Researching Health Care Consumers

Critical Approaches

Edited by

Jennifer Burr
and
Paula Nicolson

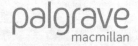
palgrave
macmillan

First published 2005 by
PALGRAVE MACMILLAN
Houndmills, Basingstoke, Hampshire RG21 6XS and
175 Fifth Avenue, New York, N. Y. 10010
Companies and representatives throughout the world

PALGRAVE MACMILLAN is the global academic imprint of the Palgrave
Macmillan division of St. Martin's Press, LLC and of Palgrave Macmillan Ltd.
Macmillan® is a registered trademark in the United States,
United Kingdom and other countries. Palgrave is a registered trademark
in the European Union and other countries.

ISBN 1–4039–0513–4

This book is printed on paper suitable for recycling and made from fully
managed and sustained forest sources.

A catalogue record for this book is available from the British Library.

10   9   8   7   6   5   4   3   2   1
14   13   12   11   10   09   08   07   06   05

Printed in China

es   rs

17.99 2
1/11/05

362.1072 Bur.

In loving memory of Mont

To Zara, Malachi and Azriel

Contents

Foreword

Elizabeth Clough

'A modern NHS is one where patients need to have power'

This quotation is not from a document produced by a 'fringe' consumer movement but from a speech by the then Secretary of State for Health, Alan Milburn, to a conference of health service managers in October, 2002.

The NHS Plan (2000) puts the patient's experience at the very heart of a modernised British National Health Service (NHS), so that services are shaped around the needs and preferences of individual patients, their families and their carers. This focuses delivery of care on consumers' needs and respects diversity in terms of age, gender, ethnicity, disability and sexuality. In 2003 a new role of Director for Patients and the Public was created in the Department of Health. The Director, Harry Cayton, will champion the voice of patients, their carers and the public in general, support staff to be responsive to the needs of patients and act as a national spokesperson in promoting the Government's patient-focused policy.

So, the policy is in place to take account of consumers' perspectives. It now needs implementation, in a comprehensive and systematic way. In order to do this a number of key questions need addressing.

What do we know already about the success or otherwise of methods of investigating the perspectives of consumers?

How do we find out what these perspectives look like and what are the philosophical and epistemological bases for different investigative methods?

What can we learn from the history of the development of the 'consumer movement' and from the experience of other public services involving their users?

These and related questions are the substance of this book.

A recurrent theme in descriptions of all the methodological approaches is the problem of the so-called 'hard to reach groups'. Evidence shows that they are under-represented amongst respondents, whatever research method is used. Of course, this group is not homogeneous and includes children, people with learning disabilities, people with dementia, some ethnic minority groups and others. It is proposed in Chapter 10 that research in the main has not tried very imaginatively to reach some of these groups. For example, visual and other methods of communication may be more appropriate than verbal. Use of information technology, discussed in Chapter 8, as well as being easier, quicker and cheaper than other methods, is also more securely anonymous and, as such, may yield higher response rates where the topic area is sensitive, for example sexual health services.

All the methods of investigation discussed – surveys by paper (Chapter 4) and telephone (Chapter 3), qualitative methods (Chapter 7), including the use of narrative (Chapter 11), methods linking preferences to economic value (Chapter 5) and Citizens' Juries and related group methods (Chapter 6) have inherent advantages and disadvantages and these are teased out. It is argued that the old chestnut – quantitative or qualitative? – is a naive and simplistic dichotomy, ultimately unhelpful in eliciting perspectives. The two complement one another and usually both are needed to support an investigation. Traditional reliance on patient satisfaction surveys frequently address the organisation's priorities rather than the consumer's; they yield overly positive results which are of little or no use in describing how to improve care. Well-constructed surveys which yield valid results are not thrown together on the back of an envelope. Similarly, the question of quality is discussed in relation to qualitative methods, which too frequently are employed with frightening lack of rigour, no demonstrable theoretical underpinning and vague, inadequate descriptions of method. In other words, talking to people and reporting a few quotations does not constitute valid evidence. With all methods it is important to acknowledge that while researchers may strive to achieve a measure of neutrality and objectivity, this can never be fully achieved. Research has a political – with a small p – element and researchers are active players, never invisible.

Social care has a 20 year history of involving users of services in the development of knowledge-based practice (Chapter 9). What counts as 'evidence' in the social care field has evolved to include service user perspectives and practitioner experiential knowledge, as well as research (scientific) knowledge. There is a frank acknowledgement of unequal power relations between professionals and consumers and a sense in which users are seen not simply as a source of data but as active shapers of knowledge and subsequent action. It seems that models of consumer involvement from social care contexts could usefully inform health research theory and practice.

Health and social care service researchers who are trying to understand and document consumers' experiences will find this book invaluable, as it offers practical advice on the pros and cons of investigative approaches. There is no such thing as 'the best method'. Enquiries may demand one method or another and frequently two or more, depending on the questions being posed. It should be read, too, by those charged with implementing the Government's policy of developing a truly patient-centred service. It is critical that those commissioning studies of consumer views of the services for which they are responsible have some understanding of what the various methods can deliver (and what they cannot).

List of Contributors

Catherine Beverley has worked as an information officer at the School of Health and Related Research (ScHARR), University of Sheffield since 2000. Here she has been responsible for providing information support and information skills training to systematic reviewers and other researchers. Prior to this she worked as a research assistant at a community NHS Trust. This included working on a project exploring the extent of consumer involvement in local research initiatives. Catherine is currently undertaking a part-time PhD exploring the health and social care information behaviour of people with a visual impairment.

Andrew Booth is Senior Lecturer in Evidence Based Healthcare Information and Director of Information Resources at the School of Health and Related Research (ScHARR) University of Sheffield. Previously he worked at the King's Fund in London where he provided information management to such projects as the 'Services for Health and Race Exchange'. His interest in evidence-based healthcare has led to his participation as expert reviewer or steering group member for several evidence-based patient information initiatives. Andrew is one of the Course Coordinators for the M.Sc in Health Informatics at the University and also teaches on the M.Sc in Health Services Research and Technology Assessment.

Steven Bruster became involved in seeking the views and experiences of patients as a researcher at St. Mary's Medical School (now Imperial College, London) during the 1990s. In 1998 he joined the Picker Institute Europe which was set up to seek the views and experiences of patients. At that time patients' views were not really taken seriously, and many managers and clinicians mistrusted the results of patient surveys. Now that patient survey results are used as part of the national performance rating within the NHS, health professionals are much more focused on this vital perspective, and the work carried out by Picker Institute Europe is taken very seriously.

Jennifer Burr has experience of qualitative research methods to investigate a range of complex issues including ethnicity and mental health, eating disorders and infertility. Having experience in also providing training for health professionals in the form of short courses on qualitative research methods and analysis she worked with busy health care professionals who were often looking for a short answer to how to conduct qualitative research and in a world where quantitative research remains the gold standard, many health carers also remain mystified at the idea that notions of validity and reliability do not apply.

This chapter reflects some of her frustrations at dealing with their frustrations.

Elizabeth Clough is in the Standards & Quality Group for Health & Social Care in the Department of Health in the UK. She became engaged with consumer involvement when she was invited to join the Consumers in NHS Research Group (now renamed INVOLVE) in 1998. For the last two years of her membership she chaired the Strategic Alliances Sub-group at a crucial time when the remit of the Group was being extended to Public Health & Social Care. In 2000/01 she was instrumental in the development of the Department of Health Research Governance Framework for Health & Social Care, the central purpose of which is to protect the research participants' dignity, rights, safety and well-being.

Some of the Medical Charities have led the way in involving consumers in active ways in health-related research and, as a member of the Multiple Sclerosis Society's Science & Development Board, she has seen at first hand how patients and carers can shape research policy.

Clare Delap became interested in public participation while completing a Master's course at the School of Oriental and African Studies, London. Public policy the world over is littered with examples of bad decisions being made by those in power because they have been unable or unwilling to involve people properly in discussion. Citizens' juries and other deliberative approaches appeared to offer one practical way to solve this crisis of dialogue and Delap has been a part of their development and use.

Shirley McIver is a sociologist by background and has worked as a health researcher for over fifteen years. She started by being involved in a project exploring the impact of the 1983 NHS Management Enquiry Report on the development of consumer feedback in the NHS, then managed a resource centre at the King's Fund that provided advice and information about getting health service users views. It was during this time that she became interested in different ways of involving patients, carers and the public in health service decisions, particularly groups which were often considered 'difficult to engage' such as people with learning disabilities and ethnic minorities.

She joined the Health Services Management Centre (HSMC), Birmingham University, UK in 1993. For the first three years this was a joint post with Premier Health Community and Mental Health NHS Trust, where she was engaged in helping the Trust to involve lay people. This included a service evaluation project with mental health service users that involved them in the research process, the training of lay associates of the Trust Board and focus group discussions with staff about developing user-centred services.

At HSMC she co-ordinates the Public and Patients as Partners in Health and Social Care Programme and runs the M.Sc./Diploma in Managing Quality in Healthcare. Activities include facilitating learning sets, developing seminars, carrying out research and consultancy, teaching and writing.

Paula Nicolson's interest in qualitative research and methods to evaluate consumer/user views of health research has different but related origins. Nicolson's interest in qualitative research per se emerged from the kinds of research questions she wanted to address: 'What is it like to be depressed?' 'How does it feel to work in this organisation?' Her interest in which methods are best able to identify the views of health care consumers came from meeting the challenge of convincing hard-line medical researchers that qualitative research questions provided data and evidence that no randomised trial could produce; which was about the experience and context of health care and what the delivery of health care in this context meant for the person receiving it. The more she works in the health research environment though, the more irritated she reports to have become with the imposition of a traditional framework for research design, data collection, reporting and analysis upon innovative qualitative methods. Nicolson chose to write her chapter in the way she has because she deplores this creeping methodolatory – or recipe book research design that many qualitative health researchers seem keen to adopt.

Alicia O'Cathain worked as a researcher in health authorities in the 1990s when they were keen to seek the priorities and preferences of their populations in response to the Local Voices initiative. She became interested in conjoint analysis as a way of engaging patients and the general population in decision-making about health services, which recognised the limited resources available to those commissioning services.

Jenny Owen is a sociologist by origin; having qualified as a teacher (adult education) in the mid-1970s, she spent 8 years working in community development and education, primarily in the voluntary sector. Her interests in ideas about users, professionals and expertise date back to her doctoral research in the 1980s; this focused on 'user-involvement' in the workplace, and specifically on women office workers' experience of information systems design and organisational change in public service contexts. Jenny's current research interests include young parents' and practitioners' differing perceptions of teenage parenthood; contrasting perspectives on 'evidence-based care' in health and social care contexts; and the role of evaluation and performance management in public services, particularly in connection with services for children and families.

Phil Shackley's interest in willingness to pay and conjoint analysis is part of a more general research interest in the area of valuing the benefits of health care for use in economic evaluations.

Graham Smith's interest in consumerism in health began in the late 1980s when he was working in Community Education with retired textile workers in Dundee. Many of the women recalled a time before the welfare state, when health care provision was inadequate for themselves and their children and that married women in the city had twice rioted in protest at the lack of benefits that condemned working mothers and their children to periodic poverty. Some years later he was given the opportunity of learning about consumerism from a different perspective when he was employed on a Wellcome History of Medicine fellowship to carry out an oral history of general practice.

Richard Wilson's involvement in this book came about as a result of work he was undertaking in research support and development on behalf of the University of Sheffield for a nearby hospital trust.

In this capacity building role Wilson had direct experience of consumer involvement in research through membership of the Trust's research governance sub-committee. It was obvious from committee discussions that for some this initiative seemed a logical extension of the general trend to increase the involvement of patients and health service users in the organisation and management of the service. For others, including Wilson, it appeared a flawed initiative driven by short term political needs where no time was allowed for a critical examination of the overall worth and value of consumer involvement.

Part One
Background

1

Critical Approaches to Researching 'consumers' of Health Care

Jennifer Burr and Paula Nicolson

Introduction

Health care organisations and health services across the industrialised world are calling for patients, service users, consumers and members of the public to feed-back their views and experiences on the quality of care, with the intention that these views will 'improve' health care. The end of the 20th and early 21st Centuries have marked the age of *participation* in health. Everyone is expected to be in a partnership. Everyone is *responsible* for their own health. The 'old' health care model, whereby the doctor provides diagnosis and a full prescription for health care delivery, has been surpassed by the rise of the role of the health care consumer. The 'consumer', 'user' (and other related terms) refer to patients, prospective patients, their carers and members of the lay communities all of whom are concerned with health. It is all of these groups and individuals involved in them who are now 'required' to take an active role in the care of their fellow citizens and themselves.

The British National Health Service (NHS) will be the main case study used throughout this book because we are writing it from a British perspective. However the NHS is experiencing a similar series of reforms to health care systems in New Zealand, Canada, Australia and other countries where there are varying degrees of socialised, or mass-insurance health care systems.

The NHS, as part of an ongoing modernisation programme, now places an increasing emphasis upon consumer 'choice' and 'empowerment' of health service users with the added implication that all aspects of health care operate from an 'evidence' or 'knowledge' base. It is the inclusion of 'consumer views' on the processes and quality of health care as part of that evidence base of effective medicine and health care delivery that is the subject of this book. How do researchers evaluate and make sense of the relationship between the delivery of health care and the experiences of those who are seeking it? People receiving health care are by definition unwell. Therefore researchers need to be able to distinguish between good quality and effective care and the health and quality of life outcomes of consumers and patients. This is a complex and potentially controversial situation to research.

In this book we assess the variability in the effectiveness of the methods through which this evidence, or knowledge, is elicited. What this book does not provide is a 'how to do research on consumers guide'. What it does provide however, is a systematic examination of the research methods currently used to evaluate the processes of health care.

The background in the UK

Successive British governments have been concerned that the NHS be more responsive to the needs and views of the public and service users (NHS Management Inquiry; Working for Patients, 1989; the Patients' Charter, 1991; NHS Management Executive's Guidance Local Voices NHSME, 1992). More recently, Government policy initiatives such as the White Paper 'The New NHS; Modern Dependable (NHS E, 1997) has placed prominence on the importance of the quality of patient experience and responding to patients' views of service. Health Authorities,

Trusts, academic researchers and consumer organisations have been attempting to emphasise the patient's perspective. A variety of research methods have been employed to elicit user views of health care. These comprise qualitative and quantitative methods including: health forums, rapid appraisal exercises, action research of initiatives in the community, public opinion surveys, patient experience surveys, one to one interviews, telephone hot-lines and focus groups.

There are two main areas that underpin the examinations of research methods presented in the following chapters. The first is the use of the concept of 'consumer' in health policy. Increasingly, health is viewed as a 'commodity' and individuals are no longer patients but 'consumers' and a key question here, which the book attempts to address, is what does 'consumer' mean in relation to health care? The second area that the book explores is the notion of 'knowledge' or 'evidence' base and what constitutes knowledge or appropriate evidence. Health policy is rooted in medical and scientific terminology and quantitative 'measurements' that can be viewed as powerful forms of rhetoric in modern society. Policy makers frequently employ this style of language believed to be most effective to convince the public of health related matters. Thus qualitative accounts have frequently lost out when policy makers cite evidence – only numbers they argue are robust. However what matters most is that whatever research is conducted it has to be done well and as part of that process the style of method should complement the research question. Whether a researcher provides numbers or words – if the design is inappropriate then the evidence is poor.

Patient as 'consumer'

The language of consumerism has become pervasive in health policy throughout the Western world reflecting a changed relationship between citizens and the state (Henderson and Petersen, 2002). The idea that the state should care for the health of its citizens is increasingly replaced by the expectation that citizens should play a more active role and have a 'duty' in caring for themselves. However, the idea that patients are consumers is contentious in spite of what can be recognised as a largely uncritical acceptance of the term in health care policy. Most authors would have few problems with the definition of 'consumer' used by Boote and colleagues (2002) as 'people who receive, or who have the potential to receive, health care' (2002, 215). However, and as Smith argues in this volume, with an emphasis upon the UK, the health care 'consumer' is a complex hybrid of policy and citizenship and has been constructed and reconstructed during the recent history of the NHS. The 'consumer' is mobilised at different times for different purposes. For example, consumerism has been used to validate policies to restrict medical autonomy (Berridge, 1999; Smith in this volume).

The rhetoric of rights and empowerment, which underpins the language of consumerism, belies the exercise of choice when many clinical encounters have a predefined and limited option for action. Furthermore, most encounters between 'consumers' and health care professionals are also governed by differentials in knowledge and therefore power. There are clearly questions on the extent to which the ideal of rational 'consumer' behaviour accords with the reality of people's everyday lives within the context of health and social care (Henderson and Petersen, 2002). This is especially the case when people are affected by conditions that involve stigmatisation, for example mental illness, they may be reluctant or unable to seek help in the prescribed ways. In a society marked by inequalities in terms of social class, gender and ethnicity one also needs to ask how relevant the 'consumer' model is. Social inequality will mark out differences with respect to expectations and definitions of need and the propensity to use services.

Writers have tended to view the term 'consumer' positively, embracing a shift from 'patient' to client' or 'consumer', as corresponding with perceived new health care citizenship and an identity label, and language for claiming rights for disadvantaged groups and challenging traditionally paternalistic characteristics of medical and health care provision. In contrast the former term 'patient' has long been recognised as representing passivity and a lack of autonomy whilst the latter implies autonomy and a 'readiness to put information to use' (Brock, 1995, 158–9). Therefore, consumerism is presented in terms of personal empowerment and freedom of choice. However, the extending reach of medicine, in terms of health promotion and mass screening programmes has helped to broaden the understanding of the 'consumer' to mean the whole population and not simply those who are ill. It has traditionally been women and children who participate in surveillance medicine but men too, are increasingly subject to surveillance schemes under the rubric of personal responsibility and the healthy lifestyle. The rise of obesity, the control of mentally ill through compulsory treatment and drug regimes, teenage parents and smokers have all come under surveillance in the interests of public health (Lupton, 1995).

The 'consumer' identity has been useful in claiming rights (for example, in the UK the battle for compensation following the prescription of thalidomide described by Smith in this volume). However, the 'consumer' label is also a means of surveillance of the population as potential health service users

What is knowledge and what is evidence?

The language of health care research is scientific and this is reflected in the gold standard of experimental design. Research in this paradigm assumes the existence of a stable reality which is independent of the observer and that an accurate observation of that reality is obtained through precise, controlled, objective observation. Experimental design is therefore, employed to isolate the variables of interest form complicating factors, and quantitative measurement are used in order to maximise the precision and objectivity of the analysis.

As Owen argues in this volume there exists a hierarchy of methods which has predominated in much health services research with research at the top which is interpreted as generating evidence based practice. However, it is our contention that there are different types of evidence, including that of 'consumer' expertise, that can be gained through different methods. The difficulty is that not all evidence is treated equally. For example, and Owen makes the case, taking social care as an example, that there are two approaches to research and the knowledge that it produces: the *empirical practice* movement, rooted in experimental designs and the second approach, *reflective practice*, allied to interpretivist and post-positivist research perspectives. Whilst it is argued that the empirical practice movement reflects a particu-

larly simplistic view of evidence, and has a tendency to decontextualise the ways in which individuals operate, this movement
continues to marginalise interpretative research approaches.
However, as Owen concludes, both the empirical practice movement and the reflective practice perspective are problematic. The
former marginalises 'consumer' expertise and whilst the latter
allows scope for dialogue, the terms of engagement are less well
defined. This dichotomy is revisited and explored in this volume,
particularly in Chapters 4 and 7.

It has certainly been argued elsewhere that 'consumer' involvement in research can result in the more subjective experiences of
patients counterbalancing clinical interests: 'when consumers'
perspectives on illness are combined with clinicians' interests in
disease, a synergistic relationship can exist and new insights can
be gained to improve the condition of the 'consumer'' (Boote et
al, 2002, 218). This is however, to assume that user and professional perspectives 'come equitably to the table' when in fact most
frequently, evidence is narrowly interpreted only as scientific.

This volume takes as its starting point the terms 'consumer' and
'evidence' as problematic. In addition, it also takes its inspiration
from and builds upon the recently completed commissioned
report[1] entitled 'Eliciting users' views of the processes of health
care: A scoping study' conducted from the University of Sheffield
School for Health and Related Research by the CHePAS team.[2]
The editors of this book are part of the original commissioned
team. The other members of the SDO team, along with other
experts, are contributors to this volume. The volume takes, as its
starting point, an assumption that the reader has a basic knowledge of research methods.

We make no claims to comprehensiveness in our presentation
of methods, perspectives and practice settings particularly given
that health care policy is constantly evolving and the extent of
involving of consumers is likely to manifest differently in different
contexts and at different times. Our aims, therefore, have been to:
a) provide a critical review of the current state of research
into 'consumer' health and consumers' views of health care;
b) provide an overview of key contemporary research methodologies used for eliciting consumer's views, with specific reference to
their strengths and limitations; c) discuss the role of the 'consumer' in health care research.

Outline of chapters

The book is divided into three sections focussing on the relevant health care policy and the emergence of the health care 'consumer', methods used in eliciting 'consumer's views and finally, critical perspectives on the limitations of 'consumer' health research.

In the Foreword Elizabeth Clough sets the policy background and includes the importance of a text of this nature in critically exploring the variety of research methods used to elicit consumers' views. Further discussion of the background is presented in Chapter 2 where Graham Smith provides an overview of the recent historical construction of the health care service 'consumer' within the UK. This includes contested definitions and representations of the 'consumer' over time. This chapter explores the emergence and development of the 'consumer' in both provider and patient perspectives.

Chapter 3 presents the results from an empirical investigation into the scope of methods used for eliciting user's views conducted for the original CHePAS project. Richard Wilson focuses upon the findings from twenty-three semi-structured telephone interviews conducted with a range of 'expert' researchers from the voluntary, health service and academic sectors. The interviews explored the respondents' experiences as researchers working in the area of consumers' views of health and health care. It outlines and discusses their views about the practice of research in this area and gaps in theory, practice and knowledge.

Wilson's chapter marks the end of the first part of the book. In the second part the reader is given a tour of different methods used in eliciting consumer's views and in Chapter 4 Stephen Bruster examines the use of survey methods. Bruster highlights the importance of a distinction between questionnaires that ask patients to rate their satisfaction and those that ask patients to report in detail on what happened to them during their health-care experience. Bruster utilises his expertise in the Picker Institute and experience in conducting the NHS Patient Survey Programme in England in making the case for quality in survey design but also offers some practical advice for readers.

There are times when we want to move beyond eliciting consumers' views towards identifying their priorities, their strength of preference for different aspects of care or for different models of service delivery, and the trade-offs they are willing to make between different aspects of care. In Chapter 5 Alicia O'Cathain and Phil Shackley summarise the literature and present the strengths and weaknesses of the techniques of conjoint analysis and willingness to pay, with a specific focus on the 'consumer'.

In Chapter 6 Claire Delap discusses the relatively new methods of citizens' juries and the deliberative family. Five years after first being piloted in the UK, citizens' juries, and other 'deliberative' approaches, have become firmly established as a mechanism for public involvement in health care decision-making. A great deal has been learned about the appropriateness of these methods and Delap discusses the circumstances in which they are most likely to be successful. However, as well as examining the features of citizens' juries and other deliberative methods Delap also considers the available evidence about outcomes and effects of deliberative approaches and asks important questions about their overall impact.

The use of qualitative methods are appraised by Jennifer Burr in Chapter 7. Qualitative methods lend themselves to eliciting users' views perhaps more than any other research methodology. However, there are real concerns in the quality of the use and reporting of qualitative methods, which are explored in detail in this chapter. Burr cautions readers against checklists for conducting qualitative research but does argue for the importance of theoretical understanding. The point is well made that we do not expect other methods to be utilised on the ad hoc basis that qualitative research methods tend to be.

Catherine Beverley & Andrew Booth consider the role of information technology (IT) in accessing 'consumer' perspectives in Chapter 8, which is also the final chapter in the methods section. IT has a valuable role to play in accessing 'consumer' perspectives. This chapter begins by analysing how technology has already been used to replace traditional methods, such as surveys, interviews and focus groups. Newer approaches (e.g. bulletin boards, electronic discussion groups, Internet chat rooms, etc.) are examined. This will be followed by an assessment of the effect of technology on the researcher-'consumer' relationship. The chapter concludes by suggesting possible methodological contributions of IT to the field of 'consumer' health research in the future.

Part Three presents critical perspectives on 'consumer' research and begins with an overview of the potential lessons which could be learnt from the UK social care context. In Chapter 9 Jenny Owen reminds us that initiatives in user and carer involvement are well-established in many areas of social care planning and evaluation. However, there is also heated debate about what constitutes valid 'evidence' in social care contexts, and about what methodological emphases are appropriate in research with and for users. This chapter provides an overview of current developments, and also examines some current and recent models of user-involvement in social care research and evaluation. In conclusion, these are placed in context with reference to the tensions and dilemmas associated with current government approaches to public sector research and evaluation.

In Chapter 10 Shirley McIver discusses some of the difficulties with 'consumer' research in that some groups and individuals remain marginalised, both in society and in research. This chapter will provide a critical overview of research methods used to examine the perspectives of users with communication difficulties. Four groups will be examined in detail: children, elderly people with dementia, people with learning disabilities and non-English speakers. The chapter will conclude with some general guidance on researching 'hard to reach' groups of service users.

Finally, in Chapter 11, Paula Nicolson examines some of the problems that qualitative researchers encounter when attempting to conduct research in a research culture that is imbued with the 'scientific' method. Attempts to ask qualitative research questions constrained in this way, has frequently led to 'lame duck' research that provides descriptions avoiding the complexities that qualitative research raises. The chapter concludes with a discussion and some examples of how well-conducted research of this kind can reveal in the context of consumers' views.

Notes

1.   Commissioned by the NHS R & D Service Delivery and Organisation
2.   Consumer Health Psychology at ScHARR.

References

Berridge, V. (1999) *Health and society in Britain since 1939*, Cambridge: Cambridge University Press.
Boote, J. et al (2002) Consumer involvement in health research: a review and research agenda, *Health Policy*, **61**(2002) 213–236.
Lupton, D. (1995) The Imperative of Health: Public Health and the Regulated Body. London: Sage.
Henderson, S. and Petersen, A. (2002) Consuming Health: The commodification of Health Care. London: Routledge.

2

The Rise of the 'new consumerism' in Health and Medicine in Britain, c.1948–1989

Graham Smith

> *... the failure to consume in due quantity and quality becomes a mark of inferiority and demerit... Conspicuous consumption of valuable goods is a means of reputability to the gentleman of leisure (Veblen, 1902).*

Introduction

A great deal of the health services research on consumerism has implied that the 'consumer' in medical and health care has only emerged as a significant figure in the last twenty-five years or so (see for example Calnan and Gabe, 2001; Boote et al, 2002). However, the 'consumer' not only appeared much earlier, but by acknowledging and exploring this history there are opportunities of understanding the ways in which the identity of the 'consumer' has been constructed and reconstructed during the recent history of health and medicine in Britain.

In the seventeenth century, 'to consume' meant to squander, to destroy, to waste and to exhaust, and then in the mid-eighteenth century the term began to be used in more neutral terms. During the eighteenth century a mutually reinforcing mixture of self-help emerged, which included the self-medication of newly available drugs for purchase, as well as the use of a range of new services (Porter and Porter, 1989). By the mid-nineteenth century the consumer had become firmly paired with the producer in descriptions of the prevailing bourgeois political economy. For some political activists consumers had become an important means of counterbalancing the power of producers. The most obvious example was the Co-operative Society's attempt to represent the interests of consumers as opposed to the interests of capital or labour. Significantly, in making this case Co-operatives directed popular political attention from the man in the workshop and towards the woman in the home. Thus, in reforming circles the growing relationship between the political economy and gender relations, capitalism and patriarchy, was recognised and even reinforced.

Around the time when the National Health Service (NHS) was founded the term 'consumer' had replaced 'customer' in economic analysis, although along the way the consumer had become gender neutral. Customer implied 'some degree of regular and continuing relationship to a supplier, whereas consumer indicates a more abstract figure in a more abstract market' (Williams, 1988, 78–9). While customers were required to be at the point of purchase and engaged in the activity of purchasing, the consumer implied a wider range of meaning, including a continuous identity with particular rights. Consumers, in contrast to customers, existed beyond the moment of purchase. And they had also started to materialise in the literature of health provision in the 1960s in Britain just at a time when 'consumerism' had begun to be more widely used, especially by sociologists (including Packard, 1961) and economists (including Godfrey, 1962) in the United States.

This chapter, beginning with the formation of the NHS, concentrates on a number of specific aspects of consumerism, including the changing relationship between the organisation and its public. After a brief survey of the early years of the institution, the nascent consumer movement is explored, including the rise of patients' and carers' organisations, from the 1960s onwards. While it is argued that this earlier history of consumerism under the NHS was patient and carer led and was concerned with empowerment of the laity, it is suggested that the more recent 'new consumerism' has its roots amongst key groups of medical and health related professionals and their response to earlier lay demands, the shifting role of the state, as well as wider socio-economic change. The result has been the dis-empowerment of both medical professionals and laity. The chapter closes with the *Working for Patients* White Paper, which not only sig-nalled the end of party political consensus in health and medical care in Britain, but was also the fanfare that announced the birth of the 'new consumerism'.

The early NHS and its public

Prior to the outbreak of the Second World War there had been a mixture of voluntary and local authority controlled hospitals and, just as in general practice, there were large geographic variations in the amount, types and quality of services that were on offer. Hospital surveys prompted by the war revealed the need for re-organisation. The charitable voluntary hospitals tended to deal with short stay cases, while the chronically sick were treated in 'unholy and unhygienic' public hospitals (Titmuss, 1950, 72) that is if they were admitted at all given the shortage of beds.

Fund raising for hospitals amongst the local communities they served was widespread, but representation on the governing bodies of these hospitals was tokenistic. Apart from a very few exceptions democratic structures and consumer involvement were absent (Gorsky et al, 2002). During the war the hospital system was nationally co-ordinated for the first time. Central planning allowed the training and distribution of professional personnel at a regional level, produced the first blood transfusion service, and initiated plans to improve dilapidated hospital accommo-dation. There was little evidence that Britain's communities thought that a loss of local control was significant. Instead, when the White Paper on *A National Health Service* was produced in 1944 'Parliament welcomed the scheme; so did almost everyone'. And as Calder adds, in a history which makes extensive use of the Mass Observation Archive, the 'chief dissenters were the leaders of the BMA' (1997, 539–40).

In both the public sphere of work and in the private sphere of the home wartime propaganda stressed the need for efficiency for the collective good. It was a point not lost on those who were arguing for an extension of national co-ordination of health and medical services. As well as the drive for efficiency there was also a growing desire that the war should create a just society. This humanitarian desire can be traced back to the nineteenth century and in particular to liberal mutualism and the co-operative movement. For many reformers, including Sir William Beveridge, the post-war welfare state was in the tradition of these earlier attempts at social amelioration. They did not see a contradiction in state provision and mutuality. Such beliefs coincided with a popular acceptance of the wartime rhetoric of egalitarianism and provided an important ideological influence in the formation of the NHS. This idealism along with the technocratic efficiency that had been born of total warfare has been described as 'a curious sort of hybrid between nineteenth century Fabian ideals and twentieth century managerialism' (Klein and Lewis, 1976, 11). This fusion, of the pragmatic and ideological, would be reinterpreted quite differently in the 1960s and again in the 1990s.

The challenges facing the new NHS were considerable. Despite the efforts of the wartime Emergency Medical Service, the NHS had inherited an incoherent and inadequate range of services. As one American commentator was to put it, 'The British have a socialised medical service simply because of the deplorable state of the old medical system' (Eckstein, 1958, 44). As well as a crumbling hospital system, severe under-investment in mental health provision, and an ageing general practitioner workforce, the NHS faced financial self-interest amongst medical professionals and resistance from planners who were reluctant to abandon local administrative practices. This was a 'flawed inheritance' (Webster, 1998, 1–64). In addition, uncertain financial planning combined with years of unmet patient demand meant that costs were rising faster than predicted. It was with a sense of regret that one of the champions of the NHS, the social scientist Richard Titmuss, reported in the late 1950s that the 'principle of free access to medical care... has to some extent been limited in recent years; primarily in respect to dental and ophthalmic care' (1976, pp. 138–9).

Concepts, such as 'consumer sovereignty', that is the belief that the use of resources is based on purchasing and that consumers ultimately determine the goods and services that are produced, were only beginning to be articulated in relation to the NHS. The Labour government had responded to Conservative fears that nationalisation would weaken 'consumer sovereignty' by establishing the Nationalised Industry Consultative and Consumer Councils, although these would make little real impact in contrast to voluntary consumerism.

In the circumstances of the immediate post-war world it is little wonder that consumer power in health provision did not feature in any meaningful way in popular consciousness. The NHS was seen by a large numbers of Britons as an important achievement; the most popular part of the welfare state. And central planning was delivering in ways that local provision had never managed. Even those historians hostile to the welfare state have acknowledged the achievements of the NHS in its early years. Lowe (1999), for example, has commended the low cost administration in comparison to services in France, Germany and the United States (p. 298). There was little sense of unease regarding the lack of consumer representation or control in the early years of the organisation. The birth of the NHS had been painful and the war-weary population was relieved that a welfare state had been established with a relatively efficient health service that was almost without charges at the point of treatment. Some contemporaries, including Richard Titmuss were however raising specific concerns. Titmuss, who served on the board of governors at Hammersmith as well as on a Regional Hospital Board, advocated democratic accountability and worried, for example, that patients' freedom to choose their doctors was too limited; a limitation forced on the Ministry of Health by clinicians in 1950 (1976, 149). Nevertheless, even Titmuss, as evident from his writings at this time, was much more exercised by the wider challenges to central planning from within the Service.

The first review of the NHS, completed in 1956, concluded that the organisation was a valuable national asset.

> *The [Conservative] Minister of Health, Mr Turton, hoped everyone would note with satisfaction, but not with complacency, that the NHS record was one of real achievement, but additional money could not be committed because of the economic situation (Rivett, 1998, 114).*

Thus began a recurring theme in the history of the NHS.

Laity, collective action and the early consumerism

In the 1960s and 1970s the state encouraged the consumer movement in health provision (Taylor, 1983, 6), with a number of the
voluntary sector pressure groups, including the anti-smoking campaign, Action on Smoking, developing close relationships with
and even receiving substantial funding from the state (Berridge,
1999, 39). The roots and development of the movement were
however more complex and would owe much to changes in the
broader meaning of consumerism and in the ideological understanding of disease and health, including within the patients'
groups themselves.

In contrast to the early state attempts to shape consumerism,
the Consumers' Association, which began testing products in a
converted garage in London's Bethnal Green in 1956, was
phenomenally successful. By the early 1960s the Association was
boasting a quarter of a million members. The then Conservative
administration responded to the birth of the Consumers' Association by setting up the Molony Committee on Consumer Protection in 1959, which led to the establishment of the Consumer
Council four years later. It was in the 1960s that the consumer, in
both state-sponsored and independent initiatives, became constructed as gender-neutral. Prior to this consumers had tended to
be portrayed as female, middle class and occupied in the home
and in the inter-war period was often assumed to be working class
housewives. Accompanying this abstraction the consumer from
the 1960s onwards was perceived not only as the 'informed' and
'discriminating' individual she had always been, but in becoming
gender neutral had also become 'efficient', 'rational', scientific',
and 'objective' (Hilton, 2003, 125–6).

Many of the political ideas expressed in the 1960s would only
begin to inform health policy much later. Conservative politicians,
for example, were attempting to find mechanisms to substitute for
consumer sovereignty as well as hoping to make the NHS fully, or
at least more fully, contributory rather than tax-funded. The
failure of this 'proto-Thatcherism' was somewhat ironically sig-
nalled by Enoch Powell, Minister of Health. Despite his leanings
towards economic liberalism, Powell's command and control
approach was expressed in his enthusiasm to make the most of
what he described as 'an opportunity to plan the hospital system

on a scale which is not possible anywhere else certainly on this side of the Iron Curtain' (cited in Lowe, 2002, 3). Powell's approach to the NHS also marked the start of a political consensus that would involve all of the major political parties and last for at least twenty years.

Amongst the incipient patients' and carers' organisations that had emerged in the early years of the NHS was the National Association of Parents of Backward Children formed in 1946 and renamed The National Society for Mentally Handicapped Children and Adults (or MENCAP) in 1963, and The Spastics Society, established in 1952, and later renamed Scope. Both organisations would prove to be influential from the 1960s onwards in their contribution to the growth of the disability movement in Great Britain. There was also a growth in the number of organisations that had begun to claim to represent health consumers more generally. These included the Association for Improvements in the Maternity Services, established in 1960, and the Patients' Association, founded in 1963.

The paternalistic welfare characteristic of the immediate postwar period was increasingly challenged with consumerism becoming a point of resistance and opposition to bureaucratic and clinical power. As the late Roy Porter noted, 'Wave after wave of protest' crashed 'against the medical system and medical establishment' (1997, 686), with powerful social critiques of medicine reinforcing lay criticisms of medical and health care orthodoxy. Concerns about the treatment and labelling of the mentally ill, had been eloquently expressed by the psychiatrist R.D. Laing (1960, 1961)[1] and the further dangers of medicalisation, including iatrogenesis, articulated by Ivan Illich (1976). As will be shown, such criticism was appearing at a time when there was increasing public dissatisfaction with conventional medicine.

Part of the reason for the transformation in public opinion was a growing disillusionment with the pharmaceutical industry and its products. In Britain one of the best-known scandals surrounded the drug thalidomide. Developed as a non-addictive sleeping pill in response to concerns surrounding barbiturates, thalidomide was prescribed to pregnant women suffering from morning sickness. Taken between the fifth and eighth weeks of pregnancy, the drug produces teratogenic effects ranging from the mild – a missing or shortened finger or two – to the extreme, including phocomelia, missing organs, and brain damage. By 1962 400 thalidomide-damaged children had been born in Britain and 10,000 world-wide. Significantly in Britain the fight for compensation lasted a decade and required a national media campaign, led by the *Sunday Times*, before the Thalidomide Children's Trust could be established in 1973 to oversee the annual allocation of the 'no blame' funds that had been won from Distillers Biochemicals. There would be other drug scandals, but few would be so protracted, involve so much publicity and would do such much damage to an individual pharmaceutical company. The health consumerism that emerged in the 1960s was shaped in part by the outrage over Distillers denials of responsibility over many years, and was accompanied by a more general loss of faith in the 'pill for every ill'.

As the power of the medical professions was being challenged by criticism and protest, there was a parallel rise in the demand for greater patient independence, with the growth of feminism playing a role in this development by encouraging patients and carers to see their health and illness in individualistic ways. In addition, the 'focus on female autonomy and self-help' would become 'part of the trend towards consumerism in health care' (Berridge, 1999, 72–3). Although seldom recognised the gender-neutral consumer of health would end up owing much to the women's movement.

By the mid-1970s the position of the medical professional in charge of health and medical care was no longer as secure as it had once been and the reputation of the pharmaceutical companies was also increasingly under threat. In response the British Pharmaceutical Industry (BPI), through its Office of Health Economics, commissioned a monograph on the possible impact of the consumer movement on the industry. The publication's author warned of a range of criticisms of the industry, including over-promotion of medicines, excessive prices, lack of safety, and the treatment of 'third world' countries. While defending the manufacturers from such charges, industry leaders were encouraged by the report's author 'to enter into dialogue with such bodies' as the 'Community Health Councils and women's organisations' (Taylor, 1983, 19–25).

The challenge from consumers to pharmaceutical multinationals, and indeed to orthodox medicine as a whole, was developing not only amongst patients' organisations, but also at an individual patient's level. And individual patients were beginning to act in ways that were much more akin to the health consumption and self-dosing, patterns of the eighteenth century by turning to alternative and complementary treatments while continuing to use orthodox medicine. By the mid-1980s the British Medical Association had become sufficiently alarmed by the growth of treatments and therapies that were outside the control of their members that they were prepared to issue an antagonistic and, given their inability to win their case, ill-thought through report in 1986. Indeed the Report rallied support for complementary and alternative medicine (CAM) and led to an increasing number of NHS doctors either referring or even practising aspects of CAM (Rivett, 1998, 381).

More visible than the rise of individualistic health behaviour was that dissent in the 1960s and 1970s had been matched by a rise in voluntarism. A survey carried out in 1978 found that almost a half of all voluntary sector organisations had been formed in the previous eight years. Groups seeking to represent the needs of patients suffering from particular diseases were amongst the fastest growing area (Finlayson, 1994, 327–8). These charities, large and small, included bodies such as the Brittle Bone Society, established as a registered charity in 1971, and the Friends of Asthma Research Council, formed in 1972. Then there was the Spinal Injuries Association (1974), The National Eczema Society (1975), the ME Society (1976), The Hyperactive Children's Support Group (1977) and DEBRA, an organisation that sought to represent people with Epidermolysis Bullosa (1978).

In 1959 Richard Titmuss had warned in a Fabian Tract that rising living standards, growing professional power and 'the acceptance of 'The Welfare State" had made 'political atheism and professional neutralism more respectable' (reprinted in Titmuss, 1976, 219–20). However, as Charles Webster the leading political historian of the NHS has subsequently argued, pressure groups, protest and criticism grew as a result of the very vacuum that had resulted from party political consensus (1998, 68). In spite of mainstream politicians, collectively the health charities represented a shift in public perceptions of voluntarism, with notions of active citizenship coming to the fore. This development bounded the growing individualism.

There were however other attitudinal changes occurring towards the NHS itself and within the voluntary organisations. The
mix of Fabianism and managerialism that had become the orthodoxy of a large part of the political spectrum meant that those
with complaints about their health and medical care, often
amongst society's most vulnerable, could, and were, often ignored
by the dominant NHS establishment. Although the patients'
organisations did not directly represent a drive by the public to be
involved in policy making, the groups did contribute significantly
to demands for patient representation and rights. For the first
time in many years the curious ideological 'hybrid' that had established the NHS was beginning to be questioned.

Attitudes towards health and medical care were also undergo-
ing an important change within the patients' and carers' organisations. This change was occurring at least in part as a result of both
generational and sectional conflicts within the charities. Younger
members, particularly of those groups that had been founded by
parents, often found themselves marginalised by a paternalistic
leadership. For example, Angela Drane, who was disabled herself,
recalled collecting for the Spastics Society and then being told by
the local non-disabled treasurer that: she 'wasn't able to count the
pennies, although I was dealing with thousands of pounds in my
local government job. It drove me mad. I left' (quoted in *The
Guardian*, 20/11/02). It would have been particularly galling for
Angela and others of her generation that the Society, like others,
had since the late 1950s been leading the campaign for the
employment of registered disabled people. The Society, along
with the other charities were the products, as well as leaders, of
their times. In many of the organisations it took a new generation
of activists to break the paternalism of the founders and to transform the 'organisations for' to 'organisations of' the disabled
(Campbell and Oliver, 1996 and Barton and Oliver, 1997).

Tensions were also present between lay and professional interests within the larger charities. These organisations were by the
1970s providing an important interface between the medical profession and members of the laity. One example that has attracted
the interest of historians is the Multiple Sclerosis Society of Great
Britain and Northern Ireland. The MS Society had been founded
in 1953 with 'very close yet deferential links with the upper eche-
lons of the medical profession'. By the mid-1970s lay deference

had turned to criticism and some of the lay members had established a patient alleviation programme and in doing so had diverted funds from the biomedical research favoured by the medical professionals. In concluding their history of the MS Society, Nicolson and Lowis (2002) have pointed out that the Society's

> ... *difficulties indicates that a degree of underlying tension between lay person and professional is structural to modern medicine and health care. In the twentieth century, orthodox medicine achieved authority and dominance hitherto unprecedented. In terms of the technical control of disease, biomedical science has made impressive strides. But its message to the laity remains essentially contradictory ... It promises cures but it must also emphasise the difficulties and limitations of medical research and medicine itself. Ultimately medicine cannot fulfil, or even adequately respond to, all of the expectations it engenders (172–3).*

Historians have also recently sought to remind us that the consumerism that exploded after decades of paternalism and silence constituted,

> *An organised social and political movement ... a genuine force for liberation for women, the working class ... as well as a set of ideas often deliberately excluded from established political organisations (Hilton, 2003).*

Even with the 'apotheosis of paternalistic rationalism, with the 1974 reorganisation of the NHS as its monument' (Klein, 1995, 95) and the lack of investment in medical and health care in the second half of the decade, the patients' groups constituted a force for change. Although the Community Health Councils, created as part of the 1974 reorganisation, can be understood as an attempt to institutionalise the consumer (Klein and Lewis, 1976), this development in itself is evidence that the voices of patients and carers were beginning to be heard.

Criticism of medical care did not mean that the idea of a government led, publicly funded, NHS had lost popular support. International context sample surveys, conducted between 1973 and 1976 in eight western countries, found that it was the British who returned the most positive evaluations of their government's role in the delivery of medical care. The Dutch, West Germans and then the Austrians closely followed (with satisfaction ranging from 78.0 to 85.3 per cent). The poorest evaluations were recorded in Italy, where 61.6 per cent of respondents reported that the government was performing badly, Finland (29 per cent) and the United States, where 38.8 per cent recorded their feelings about their government's performance in health care delivery as 'bad' or 'very bad'.

In evaluating this data, Pescosolido et al (1985) have suggested that the late introduction of public health and insurance programmes in Italy, Finland and the United States may account for their poor results in contrast to those countries with positive evaluations where health legislation had been introduced earlier. Subsequent international comparisons suggest that there is a greater degree of complexity in how public attitudes to medical and health delivery are formed than this explanation suggests. It has been argued, for example, that there is a direct correlation between higher levels of health care expenditure and higher levels of public satisfaction (Blendon et al, 1990). However, the United States, the very country where the term 'health consumer' was first coined, provides one exception to this interpretation. In the States comparatively high levels of per capita expenditure have been historically combined with low levels of satisfaction. Whatever the explanation chosen it is evident that the NHS was a robust enough institution to remain popular despite the rise of consumerism and demands for more patients' rights and autonomy, a growing critique of medical power, and a distrusted pharmaceutical industry.

Practitioners, managers, and the '*new consumerism*'

By the end of the 1970s some of the early advocates of consumerism in health were expressing reservations about the theoretical validity of the concept. The sociologist Margaret Stacey (1976), for example, pointed out that while she continued to accept that there were differences between doctors and patients they were not of a producer-consumer nature. Tudor-Hart (1995), a leading general practitioner who practised in the Welsh valleys, would later return to and develop Stacey's suggestion that patients together with their doctors were co-producers of health. The irony is that at the moment when some of the early champions of consumerism were questioning the validity of the concept in the context of health and medical care and were proposing new theoretical approaches, others of a quite different political persuasion were adopting the consumerist cause and making it their own.

The developments in the 1970s, including lay participation, would provide the basis for those who would in the next two decades attempt to fetter the power of medical professionals by 'opposing a consumer-led range of services to a professionally-led care delivery system'. This neo-liberal phase was marked, by a 'willingness of the state to attack medical autonomy and to consider a reduction of its own role' and thus represented 'significant new departures' (Lewis, 1992, 344–5). Virginia Berridge has added that,

> *The 1970s demands for increased patient power and incipient consumerism were also redefined in a new political context as the patient's rights as a consumer of health services. But consumer rights were essentially defined in a negative sense, through reduction of the power of some health care providers rather than through a positive desire to involve such 'consumers' in the running of health services and the definition of patterns of provision. This was not a democratic or collectivist vision of popular participation (Berridge, 1999, 57).*

While it is important to recognise the ways in which the political right in promoting the consumerist cause participated in the changing meaning of health consumerism, it is also valuable to separate the rhetoric of the politicians and civil servants from their actions and from the results of those actions. So, for example, in the process of attacking medical autonomy the new consumerists' plans would rest at least in part upon the sections of the medical and related professions, including general practitioners. Similarly, while aiming to reduce bureaucracy and the role of the state, a new layer of health service management would be encouraged to grow and new groups of specialist advisers would appear to support the new managerialism.

The election of the Conservative government in 1979 did not immediately mark the end of political consensus over health and medical care rather, that was to happen, as Klein (1995, 176–222) has argued, a decade later with the publication of *Working for Patients*. The first tentative steps towards changing health service provision were however being considered with aspects of the 1979 Conservative manifesto providing the basis for a new political orthodoxy. Tax relief on medical insurance schemes was restored, investment was made in the most powerful of vested interests within the NHS, the Service's structures were to be decentralised, the medical professions brought under political control, and bureaucracy was to be reduced.

By the time Thatcher had won her second term as Prime Minister there had been important structural changes in the British economy. The result of these shifts was reflected in the occupational structure, including the decline in the numbers employed in the traditional industrial sector and the rise in the numbers employed in service industries. The numbers of professionals, self-employed, and managers had increased, just as the numbers of manual workers had fallen. In 1981 non-manual workers accounted for over half of all those in waged work compared to under a third in 1951 (Price and Bain, 1988, 164). At the same time a minority of the population were finding themselves outside of the affluent society. By 1984 the unemployment rate had risen to 13.1 per cent in contrast to 1954 when the rate was closer to 1.5 per cent (Price and Bain, 1988, 174). It is hardly surprising that social attitudes in the 1980s were different from those held in previous decades. The 1980s were as far apart from the 1950s as supermarkets were from corner shops, as advertising driven conspicuous consumption by masses of individuals was from mass rationing and collective sacrifice.

While 'the revolt of the clients' (Haug and Sussman, 1969) has been recognised, the relationship of medical professionals to consumerism in health and medical care has been less well understood. Just as in other spheres active consumers have played a role in defining their own interests (Daunton and Hilton, eds, 2001), at the same time the meaning of consumerism and consumption has also been the subject of other forces and agencies. One of the most significant influences in shaping health consumerism, particular in recent decades, has been the structure of NHS itself. The division of British medicine, most notably between primary and secondary care (Honigsbaum, 1979), has shaped consumerism, especially in the last two decades of the twentieth century. While the division was neither widening nor as uniformly widespread as has often been suggested (Smith and Nicolson, 2002), relationships between general practitioners and hospital doctors have historically been difficult and by the 1990s these difficulties would lead to 'the transformation of primary care and partnerships with patients':

> *Despite and partly because of their exclusion from hospitals [soon after 1948], general practitioners discovered and explored hitherto neglected fields of effective work. Cure sometimes, comfort often, care always, in measurable terms (Hart, 1998, 1–2).*

General practice would also make a significant contribution in the construction of the new consumerism and in doing so would set itself on the path to a primary care-led NHS.

General practice was in a particularly parlous state in the first two decades that followed nationalisation of health services. GPs were widely perceived as playing a junior role to hospital based specialists, limited as they were to onward referral for all but the simplest diagnoses and treatments. Major problems had been identified in practices, problems that family doctors seemed incapable of addressing by themselves (Collings, 1950). The lack of investment in primary care along with the practitioners' insistence on independent contractor status did little to help. By the early 1960s 'as many as one in three of all new general practitioners left general practice in the UK' (Gray, 1998, 186), many of whom were emigrating. Family doctoring was proving so unattractive that predictions of its professional extinction circulated in the country's medical schools. However, it was recognised by policy makers that family doctors acting as a first point of contact reduced the numbers of patients who might otherwise seek expensive, and at the time highly valued, hospital medicine. Britain's reputation of having the greatest proportion of state-controlled medicine in the western world, while spending the smallest proportion of its GNP on health depended on the division of British medicine and general practice's gate keeping, money saving role.

In 1966 the profession secured an important material base with a new contract that had been agreed after a campaign by GPs to implement the 'Charter for the Family Doctor Service' that had been drawn up a year earlier. The contract allowed practitioners to improve premises, employ staff and encourage the further growth of group practices. There were concerns that the group practices and attached staff meant that general practitioners were 'retreating from more intimate contact with patients' (Cartwright and Anderson, 1981, 186). But the retreat would be partial and general practitioners, who consistently identified patient contact as the most rewarding aspect of their work, would remain aware of, and to some extent responsive to, rising lay demands in the 1960s and 1970s.

Family doctors remained popular with the public throughout the period (Tait and Graham-Jones, 1998, 224–5). The post-Charter generation of doctors tended to be more innovative in practice and more critical of the dominant medical culture that was so firmly based on the hospital model and drug therapies (Smith and Nicolson, 2002). As gatekeepers to secondary care they grew more comfortable in dealing with patients' complaints about hospital services and even were willing, through their College, to provide evidence to a Royal Commission in 1977 of deficiencies in their own profession's organisation of health care. Along with the growth of academic general practice in Britain's universities (Gray, 1998, 182–204), younger practitioners, as well as developing a range of new responsibilities in primary care, were also contributing to the growing critique of medical orthodoxy. Family doctors not only continued to be the first point of contact for patients, but they increasingly saw themselves at least at a practice level as providers of informed longitudinal care, which included identifying illnesses at an early stage and saving patients from the worst excesses of hospital medicine. And they could contrast their efficacy with the relatively large proportion of inappropriate clinical interventions in the United States; a country in which the clinical generalist was in rapid decline.

The renaissance of general practice in Britain included the rise of surveillance medicine in which practitioners could claim to be at the forefront of medical knowledge in screening whole populations for disease and not simply follow secondary specialists' instructions in the management of individual patients' care. The primary care practitioners who were increasingly involved in the mass screening programmes relied heavily upon the mass participation of the undiagnosed ill and healthy amongst their practice populations. Anticipatory health care including screening, health prevention (including immunisation) and health promotion, was being increasingly delivered in the community setting. By the mid-1970s Pereira Gray, an academic GP, was arguing that, 'the introduction of doctor-initiated consultations for symptom-free people has made the old definition of the word patient inappropriate' (1974, 513). Others disagreed, although forced in hindsight to recognise that preventative medicine in particular had changed the clinical relationship in primary care to such a degree that patients, even if the term was to continue to be used, encompassed a larger part of the population than previously had been the case (see for example, Marinker, 1998, 83).

This alliance of surveillance, between primary care and laity, as well as extending the reach of medicine, therefore helped to broaden the understanding of the 'consumer', to mean the entire population and not simply patients and their carers. Although, it should be noted that initially at least it was women rather than men who willingly participated in surveillance medicine. The earliest screening programmes in general practice were aimed at women and children, and it is only relatively recently that men have been subject to surveillance schemes. In addition, this change would somewhat paradoxically lay the foundations for populations to be individually charged in the future with the responsibility of producing positive health outcomes through adopting 'responsible lifestyles'.

The developing role of community medicine further encouraged general practitioners, and subsequently other primary care professionals, not only to claim a role in preventing illness developing and to protect the laity from unnecessary and inappropriate treatment, but to also assert that they were acting as patient advocates. This was in part a result of the complexity by which the hierarchy of specialist/generalist/patient was continually renegotiated in community medicine at this time (Ferguson, 2001; Fleming, 1998). The rise of patient advocacy amongst medical professionals was also an indication of the decline of lay deference. By the 1990s advocacy would extend into many more areas of health and medicine, with early development appearing in mental health provision. This spread would be identified by contemporaries as a means of 'mediating the dangers of unchecked medical paternalism' (Thomas and Bracken, 1999).

Three distinct ways of involving patients in the planning, evaluation and delivery of health care have been recognised by primary care clinicians (Pratt, 1995; Tait and Graham-Jones, 1998). In addition to the consumerist model that had developed from the lay movements of the 1960s there was said to be a 'democratic model', with Community Health Councils cited as an imperfect example. Practitioners were also keen to point out a third way, which involved patient-participation groups at practice and local area levels. First developed in Oxfordshire in the 1970s (Pritchard, 1981), these groups were forerunners of a raft of bodies that would at the turn of the century become anointed representatives of the health consumer.[2] This was particularly the case in England, where in the devolved NHS the extinction of more democratic organisations, such as the Community Health Councils, has yet to be fully regretted.

By the 1980s Conservative politicians had identified general practice as a key to the implementation of its policy aims. The arguments for a primary care NHS, especially the cost-saving argument that secondary care treatment was more expensive than health promotion and illness prevention programmes in primary care, had been taken up by an alliance of civil servants and a growing band of health economists.

From the earliest days of their sub-discipline health economists had been interested in 'consumer choice' (see for example Lees, 1961). Emerging as a sub-discipline in the 1970s, the leading 'academic entrepreneurs' at York's Health Economists' Study Group (HESG) forged links with those civil servants responsible for the NHS (Croxson, 1998). Together they aimed to refashion the consumer, who, while remaining rational and informed, would become a partner of providers and the purchasers of provision. Thus the 'econocrats' produced 'a new form of [Benthamite] rationalism' in which 'inefficiency and ignorance' were denounced 'as the ultimate sins' (Klein, 1995, 194). In doing so they also redefined the meaning of efficiency, by narrowing an earlier understanding that 'waste' could be thought of in social and not simply fiscal terms, and knowledge, by insisting that it was through health economics that the problems of the NHS could be both identified and solved.

While proclaiming their hostility to bureaucracy, successive Conservative governments found themselves responsible for a NHS in which the power of the manager and planner actually increased. In particular, the Griffiths Report (1983) 'led to sweeping away of consensus management teams and their replacement by general management' (Webster, 1998, 40). And yet the Report also provided the rhetoric and expectations that there would be a shift of power from providers to consumers. In the next decade the increasing introduction of market conditions in the name of the consumer would be accompanied by increasing managerialism.

The practitioners' surveillance role was identified as especially significant by the econocrats and right-wing politicians, especially the 'rhetoric of prevention' which became 'harnessed to the cause of cost control' (Lewis, 1992, 342). At the same time GP fundholding was increasingly seen as a way of introducing an internal market into the NHS. By the late 1980s promises were being made that fundholding would provide patients with an increased choice of available services. The general practitioner would become the consumer's representative and consumers would be able to change their practitioner if they did not approve of her or his use of NHS resources on their behalf. However, there was little evidence that patients would shop around (Lewis, 1998, 143), that the arrangement would result in consumers driving the NHS, or that most GPs would act as entrepreneurs even though they had retained independent contractor status. Rather it was the purchasers, fundholding general practitioners along with Health Authorities, who would become proxy consumers (Klein, 1995, 191). And, as one contemporary policy observer put it, the agenda seemed to include replacing the 'paternalism of the doctor' with 'the paternalism of the manager' (Paton, 1992, 122).

In 1990 a new contract was imposed on general practice, specifying the services that they would provide. The contract offered to meet many of the demands that GPs had been making, including being able to conduct minor surgery. However, they feared, quite correctly as it turned out, that there would be an increase in their administrative workload and that they would find themselves operating in an overly bureaucratically and complex system in which easily measured work, regardless of clinical value, would be rewarded (Lewis, 1998, 143–4).

Along with the new GP contract and, as already noted, the *Working for Patients* White Paper (1989) proved to be the precursor to a host of changes that have taken place in the NHS in recent years. However, these changes were not simply a result of a chance comment by a Prime Minister on a television programme, or even a government that with a third election victory was more confidently pursuing its market minded ideology, or even a government faced by expanding demand in health while committed to containing public expenditure (Klein, 1995, 176). Rather these changes were planned and implemented in a NHS that was already being shaped by a range of different forces, including greater public awareness of health and medicine that had resulted from the earlier consumerism movement, the long rise of both general practice and the more recent emergence of the econocrats.

Conclusion

The consumerism that developed in the 1960s and onwards was a political movement that developed amongst patients and carers and challenged the existing medical orthodoxy. While parts of this movement were supported by the state, consumerism was neither state sponsored nor government designed to the extent that it became in the 1980s and 1990s. In arriving at this conclusion it is worth noting that it is an exaggeration that, 'Dying has become the ultimate form of consumer resistance' as the editor of the British Medical Journal suggested in a review of the work of Ivan Illich (2002, 923). There would be a new wave of campaigning groups that would emerge in the mid-1990s, most notably around HIV/AIDS, and that these might be considered the 'fourth estate' in medicine (Allsop, 1995, 254). However intervening social and political changes, including the demise of political consensus over the NHS itself and the rise of individualistic health consumption, meant that these organisations did not represent the radical challenge that their predecessors had. Indeed, while the earlier movement might be described as empowering patients, carers and the laity more generally, the later promotion of consumerism by the political right not only reduced medical autonomy, but also ensured that the 'new consumers' have fewer opportunities of demanding a democratically accountable NHS.

The rapid development of a radical critique of medicine in the 1960s and 1970s was matched by a growth in individualism in popular understandings of health and medical care, which would provide within the context of wider socio-economic changes the beginnings of the demise of more collective perspectives. The critique developed not only amongst intellectuals like Illich, but also amongst patients, their carers, and rank-and-file health professionals especially those who were working in community settings. The seeds of the 'new consumerism', which included using individual aspirations to limit medical autonomy, are therefore to be found in the earlier history. However, the history of the earlier period also suggests that even in the midst of party political consensus new ways of understanding relationships in health and medical care can rapidly emerge. These developments will accelerate as local democracy is re-strengthened. So, for example, under devolution, there are signs of new lay-professional partnerships beginning to be established in Scotland and Wales.

The pharmaceutical industry has recovered much of its reputation since the years of the thalidomide scandal, but there are signs that the industry is coming under renewed criticism, for example in the charge that pharmaceuticals are currently engaged in 'disease mongering' (Moynihan et al, 2002). And complementary and alternative forms of medicine have gained a greater foothold in health and medical provision. It was estimated that by 1995 over 39 per cent of all general practices were providing access to complementary therapies for their NHS patients with around 10,000 patients per week being referred to CAM practitioners (Thomas et al, 2001). While the tensions between orthodox and alternative therapies may have eased, an understanding of the recent past would lead to the conclusion that this is a temporary truce that may be broken as orthodox medicine continues to promise much more than it can deliver, even if it incorporates elements of CAM.

It has been argued by policy makers that under the new consumerism 'patients are expected to want more choice in future and to demand higher quality services' (Wanless, 2002, 14). At the same time studies also suggest a growing 'social segregation and polarisation, between the prosperous majority and those who depend entirely on public services' (Mohan, 2003, 11). A new social arrangement seems to be emerging, especially in England, with the taxpaying majority having to be reassured that they can obtain a high quality service by shopping around, and, it is hoped, that by being reassured as consumers they will continue to be bound to the welfare state as taxpayers. Recent research also suggests that there is only a small proportion of the UK population with private health insurance (around 12 per cent), but that the proportion is much higher in those key constituencies in which Labour secured victory in 1997 and again in 2001. It seems that there are some patients who count for much more than others in the new political consensus.

While patient surveys suggest that the NHS has historically retained public support, there are grounds for caution. So, for example Mossialos (1997) has noted that respondents in the UK appeared to be more favourably inclined towards a major reform of the system than is the case in other European countries. In addition, there was a great deal of pessimism expressed about the quality of future health care and ability to pay for new developments out of the public purse. Such evidence provides hope not only for those who support an extension of the NHS ethos, but also to those who are intent on the further introduction of market forces. There are already warning signs that the World Trade Organisation is attempting to force governments to open up their public services to multinational service providers. In doing so those health-care systems that guarantee access to health and medical care as a universal right will come under threat (Pollock and Price, 2000).

Notes

1.   Laing's *Self and Others* (1961) was republished by Penguin in 1971 and *The divided self* (1960) was republished by Penguin in 1976.
2.   The National Institute of Clinical Excellence, for example, established a Citizens Council in 2002 to assist in deciding on how clinical need should be judged.

References

Allsop, J. (1995, 2nd edn) *Health policy and the NHS. Towards 2000*, London: Longman.
Baker, A. (ed.) (2000) *Serious shopping, psychotherapy and consumerism*, London: Free Association Books.
Barton, L. and Oliver, M. (eds) (1997) *Disability studies: past, present and future*, Leeds: Disability Press.

Berridge, V. (1999) *Health and society in Britain since 1939*, Cambridge: Cambridge University Press.

Boote, J. et al (2002) Consumer involvement in health research: a review and research agenda, *Health Policy*, 61(2002) 213–236.

Blendon, R.J., Leitman, R., Morrison, I. and Donelan, K. (1990) 'Satisfaction with health systems in ten nations', *Health Affairs*, Summer, 185–192.

Boote, J. et al (2002) Consumer involvement in health research: a review and research agenda, *Health Policy* 61(2002) 213–236.

Calder, A. (1997) *The people's war: Britain 1939–1945*, London: Pimlico.

Calnan, M. and Gabe, J. (2001) 'From consumerism to partnership? Britain's national health service at the turn of the century', *International journal of health services*, 31(1), 119–132.

Campbell, J. and Oliver, M. (eds) (1996) *Disability politics: understanding our past, changing our future*, London: Routledge.

Cartwright, A. and Anderson, R. (1981) *General practice revisited: a second study of patients and their doctors*, London: Tavistock Publications.

Collings, J.S. (1950) 'General practice in England today: a reconnaissance', *Lancet*, i. 555–85.

Croxson, B. (1998) 'From private club to professional network: an economic history of the Health Economists' Study Group, 1972–1997', *Health Economics*, 7, Supplement 1, S9–S45.

Daunton, M.J. and Hilton, M. (eds) (2001) *The politics of consumption: Material culture and citizenship in Europe and America*, Oxford: Berg.

Eckstein, H. (1958) *The English health service*, Harvard: Harvard University Press.

Ferguson, R. (2001) 'Autonomy, Tension and Trade-off: attitudes to doctors in the history of district nursing', *The International History of Nursing Journal*, 6(1).

Finlayson, G. (1994) *Citizen, State and Social Welfare in Britain, 1830–1990*, Oxford: Clarendon Press.

Fleming, V. (1998) 'Autonomous or automatons? An exploration through history of the concept of autonomy in midwifery in Scotland and New Zealand' *Nursing Ethics: an International Journal for Health Care Professionals*, 5(1): 43–51.

Godfrey, S.E. (1962) *Retail Selling and Organization. A survey of modern methods in retail distribution, etc.* London: Cassell.

Gorsky, M., Powell, M. and Mohan, J. (2002) 'British hospitals and the public sphere: contribution and participation before the NHS'. In Sturdy, S. (ed.) *Medicine and the public sphere in Britain, 1600–2000*, London: Routledge, pp. 123–45.

Gray, D.J.P. (1974) 'What is a patient?', *Journal of the Royal College of Practitioners*, 24, 513.

Gray, D.J.P. (1998) 'Postgraduate training and continuing education', in Loudon, I. et al (eds), 182–204.

Hart, J.T. (1995) 'Clinical and economic consequences of patients as pro-ducers', *Journal of Public Health Medicine*, 17(4) 383–6.

Hart, J.T. (1998) 'Our feet set on a new path entirely: To the transforma-tion of primary care and partnership with patients', *British Medical Journal*, 317(7150), 1–2.

Haug, M.R. and Sussman, M.B. (1969) 'Professional autonomy and the revolt of the customer', *Social Problems*, 17(2) 153–161.

Hilton, M. (2003) *Consumerism in twentieth century Britain: The search for a historical movement*, Cambridge: Cambridge University Press.

Honigsbaum, F. (1979) *The division in British medicine: a history of the sepa-ration of general practice from hospital care 1911–1968*, London: Kogan Page.

Illich, I. (1976) *Limits to medicine. Medical nemesis: the expropriation of health*, London: Calder and Boyars.

Klein, R. and Lewis, J. (1976) *The politics of consumer representation*, London: Centre for Studies in Social Policy.

Klein, R. (1995, 3rd edition) *The new politics of the NHS*, London: Longman.

Laing, R.D. (1960) *The divided self*, London: Tavistock Publications.

Laing, R.D. (1961) *Self and others, Further studies in sanity and madness*, London: Tavistock Publications.

Lees, D. (1961) 'Health through choice', Hobart Paper 14, Institute of Economic Affairs.

Lewis, J. (1992) 'Providers, 'consumers' the state and the delivery of health care services in twentieth century Britain'. In Wear, A. (ed.), *Medicine in society*, Cambridge: Cambridge University Press, pp. 317–45.

Lewis, J. (1998) 'The medical profession and the state: GPs and the GP Contract in the 1960s and the 1990s', *Social Policy and Administration*, 32(2) 132–50.

Loudon, I. et al (eds) (1998) *General practice under the National Health Service, 1948–1997*, Oxford: Oxford University Press.

Lowe, R. (1999, 2nd edn) *The welfare state in Britain since 1945*, Basingstoke, Macmillan.

Lowe, R. (2002) 'Financing health care in Britain since 1939', *History and Policy*, http://www.historyandpolicy.org/archive/policy-paper-08.html.

Marinker, M. (1998) ''What is wrong' and 'How we know it': Changing concepts of illness', in Loudon, I. et al (eds), 65–91.

Mossialos, E. (1997) Citizens' Views on Health Care Systems in the 15 Member States of the European Union, *Health Economics*, 6: 109–116.

Moynihan, R. et al (2002) 'Selling sickness: the pharmaceutical industry and disease mongering', *British Medical Journal*, 324, 886–891.

Mohan, J. (2003) *Reconciling equity and choice? Foundation Hospitals and the future of the NHS*, London: Catalyst.

Nicolson, M. and Lowis, G.W. (2002) 'The early history of the Multiple Sclerosis Society of Great Britain and Northern Ireland: A sociohistorical study of the lay/practitioner interaction in the context of a medical charity', *Medical History*, 46, 141–174.

Packard, V. (1961) *Waste makers: On American methods of stimulating industrial consumption*, London: Longmans.

Paton, C. (1992) *Competition and planning the NHS: the danger of unplanned markets*, London: Chapman Hall.

Pescosolido, B.E., Boyer, C., Tsui, W.Y. (1985) 'Medical Care in the Welfare State: A Cross-national Study of Public Evaluations', *Journal of Health and Social Behaviour*, 26, 276–297.

Pollock, A.M. and Price, D. (2000) 'Rewriting the regulations: how the World Trade Organisation could accelerate privatisation in health-care systems', *The Lancet*, 356(9246), 1995–2000.

Porter, D. and Porter, R. (1989) *Patient's progress: doctors and doctoring in eighteenth century England*, Oxford: Polity.

Posnett, J. (1999) 'Is bigger better? Concentration in the provision of secondary care', *British Medical Journal*, 319, 1063–1065.

Pratt, J. (1995) *Practitioners and Practice: A Conflict of Values?* Oxford: Radcliffe Medical Press.

Price, R. and Bain, G.S. (1988) 'The labour force'. In Halsey, A.H. (ed.) *British social trends since 1900: a guide to the changing social structure of Britain*, London: Macmillan.

Pritchard, P. (1981) 'Patient participation in general practice', RCGP occasional paper, 17.

Rivett, G. (1998) *From cradle to grave. Fifty years of the NHS*, London: King's Fund.

Smith, G. and Nicolson, M. (2002) An oral history of everyday general practice: Beyond the practice: the changing relationship with secondary care, *British Journal of General Practice*, 52(484), 956–7.

Smith, R. (2002) 'Limits to medicine. medical nemesis: The expropriation of health – a review', British Medical journal, 324, 923.

Stacey, M. (1976) 'The Health Service consumer: a sociological misconception', in Stacey, M. (ed.) *The sociology of the National Health Service: Sociological Review*, monograph 22.

Tait, I. and Graham-Jones, S. (1998) 'General practice, its patients, and the public', in Loudon, I. et al (eds), 224–46.

Taylor, D. (1983) The consumer movement, health and the pharmaceutical industry, London: Office of Health Economics.

Thomas, K.J., Fall, M. and Nicholl, J. (2001) 'Access to complementary medicine via general practice', *British Journal of General Practice*, 51, 25–30.

›Thomas, P.F. and Bracken, P. (1999) 'The value of advocacy: putting ethics into practice'. *Psychiatric Bulletin*, 23, 327–329.

Titmuss, R.M. (1950) *Problems of social policy*, London: HMSO.

Titmuss, R.M. (1976, 3rd edn.) *Essays on 'the welfare state'*, London: George Allen and Unwin.

Veblen, T (1902) *The theory of the leisure class: an economic survey of institutions*, New York: Macmillan.

Wanless, D. (2002) 'Securing Our Future Health: Taking a Long-Term View; Final Report', HM Treasury, http://www.hm-treasury.gov.uk/Consultations_and_Legislation/wanless/consult_wanless_final.cfm

Williams, R. (1988, 2nd edition), *Keywords: A Vocabulary of Culture and Society*, London: Fontana Press.

Webster, C. (1998) *The National Health Service: a political history*, Oxford: Oxford University Press.

Webster, C. (1998) 'The politics of general practice', in Loudon, I. et al (eds), 20–44.

3

'You have to be pragmatic' Methods, Epistemology and Consumer Involvement in Research

Richard Wilson

Introduction

The purpose of this chapter is to develop further some findings from a study undertaken originally for the NHS Service Delivery and Organisation agency, that examined and evaluated research methods used to elicit health service users' views of the processes of health care, particularly focusing on the efficacy of these methods. In addition, the investigation aimed to identify gaps in the overall knowledge base. The original part of the study reported here ('Eliciting Users' Views of the Processes of Health Care: A Scoping Study' 2001)[1] was based upon the analysis of interview material gathered from 23 different individuals[2] who occupied a variety of positions in a range of key organisations and agencies, all with acknowledged expertise in methods for eliciting users' views of health care.

This chapter focuses on the four main themes: 1) the quality of the knowledge base concerning user involvement; 2) the paucity of published material on this topic; 3) issues around resourcing research in this area; and 4) the ongoing debate about the most appropriate research method to use.

It is argued that there are some misguided assumptions made about the use of user/consumer views about the processes of care and the research that apparently highlights these views may be misguided.

The means and methods of carrying out these interviews are detailed here at the end of this chapter.

Findings from the interviews

1) The quality of the knowledge base concerning user involvement

> 'I'd like to see how consumer views are being used effectively to change practice with examples' (NHS researcher).

The drive to widen participation in the research process has been an established part of government policy since 1991 (Blaxter, 1995). Too often in the past, so the argument runs, health research was an activity engaged in by professional researchers for their own specific purposes. These purposes may have had little or no relevance to the health service users or to those who actually fund that research. However, by bringing in the consumers of care (and ultimately consumers of the products of research), the quality of the research and also its utility are expected to improve. The problem though, is *that evidence of this assertion is hard to come by* making it difficult to convince sceptics that there is any value to consumer involvement. Many of the participants in this project commented on the need for more research-based assessments of user involvement being placed in the public domain. These would provide the details of how and in what situation users had been successfully or not involved in the research process. That these pieces of research are lacking such detail seriously undermines the whole case. For example:

> 'There is actually very little research that you can use to prove that user involvement is worth doing and I think that's the biggest gap in research. Certainly for

us if you're trying to convince people who think evidence base is the important thing to look at and you don't have an evidence base, it's bloody difficult actually. Something that you could wave under people's noses, doctors particularly, to say 'Look, here's the evidence that it's worth spending time on because we know it's time consuming, it's costly, it's not easy;' and you could say to people we know those things but we can see it does definitely make services better or more appropriate or whatever it does. That for me is the biggest gap in research' (academic researcher).

This neatly illustrates the theoretical and methodological problems with 'consumer' involvement in research. Firstly, there is the problem that little research is being undertaken on the topic and therefore a corresponding sparseness in evidence for the utility of the movement as a whole: '*There is very little research that you can use to prove that user involvement is worth doing*'. In other words this is a politically driven initiative which has largely failed to attract substantial research interest, or, where it has attracted interest, the projects have not generated data that supports the initiative. Secondly, the absence of this evidence base means that convincing others who are initially sceptical may become a challenge. '*If you're trying to convince people who think evidence base is the important thing to look at and you don't have an evidence base, it's bloody difficult*'. However, and particularly interesting, is that this academic researcher still remains convinced about the necessity of involving consumers: '*we can see it does definitely make services better or more appropriate or whatever it does.*' It was evident in many interviews that the involvement of consumers, in spite of an acknowledged lack of evidence, has become an article of faith; consumer involvement is worthwhile even when interviewees were unable to point to any 'scientific' justification.

However, the question of what constitutes acceptable 'evidence', as discussed throughout this book is crucial. Even when researchers felt that they had established an 'evidence-base', those who were in a position to change practice did not always recognise it. For example, one researcher argued:

'*What happened when we tried to implement the findings was when it came down to a particular ward they would say, 'well, we're not sure whether this is applicable to us. If 72 per cent of patients said verbal communication with doctors was poor then that's not the case on our ward*' (researcher in the health service).

The question about what might or might not constitute an evidence-base has serious practical and theoretical implications for researchers and the involvement of health service users. As one researcher stated: *'There is a tendency for professionals to stamp on users and say that's just anecdotal and it's a question of what kind of evidence you're going to consider'*. The use of the expression 'anecdotal' appears to have implications about the value of qualitative research with the hidden suggestion that qualitative research may not yield evidence that is considered appropriate for health care professionals. This same researcher goes on to argue:

> *'You shouldn't undermine what people say, and that happens a lot. You also need to choose lay representatives carefully. They need to have personal and social skills to be able to participate effectively. You also need at least two users as they are often working against entrenched clinicians or professionals who are often seeped in grades of evidence' (academic researcher).*

The key phrase here is 'seeped in grades of evidence'. It is a recognition by the speaker that clinicians operate within a positivist, quantitative, paradigm that actively discriminates against utilising or accepting data that originates from within an alternative research approach. No doubt qualitative research as one of those alternative approaches occupies the bottom end of the grades of evidence referred to. As do, it would appear, those who rely on it. The discrimination extends beyond the issue of research paradigm to include the social attributes of consumer representatives and their acknowledged inability to speak the same language as the medical professionals. The implications for marginal groups, e.g. people with disabilities, mental illness or those for whom English is not their first language, is that they are already discounted and that their views do not count (see also Chapter 10).

Participants from the voluntary sector had a different view of the evidence problem. Who benefits from research into user views? Much research lacked value for users as there was a differing perception of how a useful outcome to a project might be defined. For voluntary sector representatives evidence was seen to be less as 'published output' and more as concrete 'achievements in service delivery'. The problem here, as they articulated, was that despite apparently 'never-ending research', and requests for nominal assistance or involvement in that research, no obvious changes or benefits were ever discerned. This dispiriting state of affairs leads to 'user fatigue'. One representative expressed it as: '*People get really fed up about being asked the same questions in different ways over and over again and never seeing any difference to the way care is provided*'. Another voluntary sector representative echoed this sentiment:

> '*I mean, I must say I get two questionnaires a week from somebody or other, you know, university researchers, researching say the voluntary sector and they all assure me that somehow in some vague way I or my organisation will benefit fantastically from my filling in their questionnaire and sending it back to them. But I have to say I'm rarely convinced and I rarely do it*' (voluntary sector representative).

It would appear then that there is a gap between what is recognised as knowledge and then getting that knowledge implemented. While professionals may question what constitutes a knowledge base, with the implication that only socially skilled users can provide appropriate evidence, it is users of services who remain in a vacuum and are not benefiting from the research they are being asked to participate in.

2) *The paucity of published material on this topic*

'*There is no time to write stuff up…*' (NHS researcher)

A further problem identified by the researchers who participated in this study was the quantity and quality of published papers that are available in the area of users' views. While innovative and creative practice was presumably being undertaken it wasn't being written up, published or disseminated in an effective way. As one academic researcher stated:

> '*There is no time to write stuff up [...] and good research never getting into the public domain with bits that never saw the light of day and never got written up because it got marginalised (within the research).*' (academic researcher)

There are multiple reasons for this. As the researcher quoted above has argued, publications do not always focus upon methods, particularly what has gone wrong or required inventive measures.

There is also a tension between the need to focus on what is practical or achievable and the perception of journals as being preoccupied with a theoretical debate about methods. As one academic researcher stated: '*You have to be pragmatic about what's going to work with your particular group, not with what's been written up in* Social Science and Medicine *really.*' (academic researcher). The difficulty exposed in these interviews is that if methods and findings are not peer reviewed the process of gathering knowledge and therefore the knowledge itself is not open to scrutiny and critical debate and the wider community of researchers (together with users of health services) do not have the opportunity to learn from the process. However, other researchers highlighted different reasons for this, which varied across the organisations consulted. For example, those working for charities, NHS trusts and organisations located outside of universities had limited time to write research papers. This was also true for some university research staff who had short-term contracts and therefore had to move from project to project without time to write for publication.

Overall, there is little evidence to suggest that these researchers are making a determined effort to grapple with the multi-faceted nature of social life and develop a clear line of reasoning for their research strategies. They seem instead content to wallow in a sea of epistemological and ontological uncertainty, grasping at whatever pragmatic pieces of methodological flotsam come within reach.

3) Issues around resourcing research in this area

'You can't just do it on a shoe string.' (health-service based researcher)

Interviewees were concerned to point out that research costs money regardless of whether or not that particular piece of research involves the use of consumers. Naturally, there is a problem for all researchers in obtaining funding but the feeling among the respondents is that insufficient recognition is given to the additional costs incurred in organising research where consumers are involved. The health researcher quoted at the head of this section also stated that, '*if you're going to do things properly it does cost money*'.

Designing and implementing research projects where consumers are central is not a cheap option. Respondents argued
that funding bodies appeared to think that consumer involvement
can be 'bolted on' to a project design without any great difficulty.
However, as one respondent stated:

> 'You've got to ensure there's the resource and capacity to support people because
> the time it takes people, just needs so much time, not only needing regular corre-
> spondence and feedback and communication. I mean, I can spend hours, not
> hours, but at the beginning a lot of my time was taken up with calls and things
> and it's got added to my job. So, it's really difficult, so it's not a full-time job but
> it could easily be' (researcher, voluntary sector).

As this respondent says, a great deal of time and effort has to be
put into finding the consumers and then involving them in a
meaningful way. It requires a specific approach to project design
and construction with time being made available for first eliciting
and then subsequently making some effective use of the consumer input. Planning for user involvement needs to be prospective, not retrospective, and proper account has to be taken of the
labour involved. As one researcher interviewed stated, '*They
[funders] could think more about properly resourcing it*'.

4) *The ongoing debate about the most appropriate research method to use*

'*...you have to be pragmatic...*'

Flexibility is an essential attribute for a researcher. Research, like
life generally, rarely proceeds exactly according to plan. Pragmatism, in the sense of not being rigidly bound to a particular
paradigm or perspective is a virtue to be lauded. Unfortunately,
for these respondents, a preoccupation with pragmatism appears
to be as much a cloak for the lack of coherence in their epistemological base as it is indicative of a flexible and open-minded
attitude.

The problem is illustrated by one researcher who said, '*...it's
about finding which methods work in which situation.*' It is indeed a
question which needs to be asked and as hinted earlier in the

chapter there is a tension between the apparent scientific acceptability of positivistic, quantitative, methods and qualitative approaches which would allow the actual voice of the research
participant to be heard clearly.

Aspects of this debate are echoed throughout this book.
Nevertheless, the debate is particularly apposite when considering
the involvement of 'consumers' in research. Is there, in this particular case, some factor so intrinsically different or problematic
about research involving consumers that it requires a methodological debate of its own? The question remains unanswered.
However, it was recognised that, *'The weakness of nearly all the
methodologies is that it's quite difficult to reach the inarticulate or disem-
powered consumer.'* (voluntary sector representative). As discussed
earlier respondents did recognise that there were certain groups
to whom this might apply – the frail elderly, the young, those with
poor literacy, disabilities, and users and carers living in rural
settings (see Chapter 10).

In the meantime though the researchers quoted here are left
with the real dilemma that for this type of research there really is
no clear indication about whether qualitative or quantitative
methods are best suited to this research. Earlier it was noted that
researchers reflected upon the lack of published material that was
available to them. One of the consequences of having no literature to refer to is the sense of isolation that can develop and the
researcher's inability to even begin to resolve epistemological
debates of this kind.

For some respondents though there was an overly pragmatic air
to their approach. It is not that one needs to engage in methodological novelty (or experimentation), it is more a simple matter
of sticking with what works: *'I don't think it's about finding new
methodologies. I think it's about finding which methods work in which situations.'* One academic researcher put it as, *'just thinking beyond the
normal barriers [...] so you can twiddle with the techniques.'* So perhaps
there is no need for novelty or innovation in this kind of research,
more the open-minded acceptance that anything might possibly
work and that therefore anything is worth trying. As another
researcher stated, *'Clearly what you need is a plurality of methods.'* It is
an attractively simple thought although perhaps naïve when one
considers the complex ontological and epistemological assumptions that ultimately lie behind the adoption of a research

method. In addition there is the tension identified above between the idea that the choice of methods must, by necessity, be driven by pragmatic considerations rather than by an informed episte-mological and ontological understanding of how and why a par-ticular method might be applicable. But if one is going to go for a plurality of methods it would be well to cover the 'newer' methods such as citizens' juries, health panels, patient forums (all methods which are dealt with in this collection) and patient stories or diaries. A number of respondents indicated their interest in these less orthodox methods.

The absence of a secure methodological grounding has adverse consequences for the research that is carried out. A pressing issue of concern identified by one health services researcher was the quality of research that was being undertaken by researchers.

> *'I get calls all the time from people in trusts saying they want to do a focus group with, say, cancer patients and haven't done one before. Because it's the flavour of the month they think they can, with a couple of hours talking people on the phone, they can walk into a group and run one. So you need to think carefully about who runs them, and having others there to help run it. Again, that has cost implications.' (researcher in the health service).*

So there are, according to this researcher, profound implications for the quality of the work that is undertaken by health profes-sionals with no formal training or expertise in research methods. The end result is that, *'People do shoddy, shoddy, work which hurts patients and is unethical. Now it's done under the quality management, clinical audit banner so someone will say I'm doing an audit. There's no explanation of how it was going to be used, what it's for, or how they get their name and address.'* (researcher in the health service)

Conclusion

The interviews reanalysed for this chapter revealed that researchers in the field are confronted by many problems when facing up to incorporating the views of consumers into their research. The problems encountered are inter-related and have a tendency to work synergistically, thus compounding the overall effect. There is primarily no evidence that researchers can call upon when developing projects to guide them in selecting designs that are effective or that work well. At a time when evidence based practice is promoted as the panacea for all ills the consumer oriented researcher finds that for this branch of research there is no knowledge or evidence base. In part this must be due to the acknowledged lack of relevant published material. Whatever is happening, whether good or bad, it isn't making it into the public domain. This may be because the researchers concerned are particularly shy and shun the public spotlight or alternatively because they are held back by other factors. One factor given explicit mention was the time involved to prepare the written academic output from a project. Securing a publication would be the logical and desirable endpoint but one that seems completely absent here as no-one has thought to plan for it. Again, this is a partial consequence of the non-existent knowledge base. Without any firm evidence or guidance on good project design and the additional demands that this type of research places on those who engage in it, it becomes difficult to communicate to the bodies that are commissioning and funding the research that space needs to be built into the project for consumer involvement (and also to adequately publicise the methodological lessons to be learned). It is in practical terms a resource issue but one that is unrecognised and, tautologically, difficult to justify when there is no evidence that highlights the importance of publication and thus knowledge creation. Finally, researchers discover that they are in a paradigmatic wilderness where all and any research methods or techniques can be considered valid or at least worth a try. It is refreshingly pragmatic but as an approach it runs the risk of researchers drifting off into a state of methodological anomie.

Postscript on the methods

Contacting respondents

Key individuals, all known for their work and expertise in methods for eliciting user views, were purposively selected as potential participants for interview. This group of people comprised individual researchers drawn from organisations conducting research and evaluation studies, consumer representative groups and health service professionals. To widen the interview cohort a 'snowballing' technique was pursued with the initial group being asked to suggest further organisations or individuals that they considered pivotal in this area. Following this, in October 2000, letters were sent to all those who had been identified inviting them to participate in the study. A follow-up telephone call was made a week later to establish whether or not the person was willing to participate and also to provide more detailed information about the study than had been contained in the initial mailing. The project protocol originally called for all respondents to be interviewed 'face to face' but owing to a tight schedule the majority of those taking part were interviewed by telephone.

All of the individuals who were contacted by the research team with a request for their participation did agree to take part. Prior to the interview proper each respondent received by post or e-mail a copy of the interview guide in order that they might have time to think about the questions and the content of their answers. A breakdown of the respondents' backgrounds show that thirteen were drawn from academic organisations, four came from the service user/voluntary sector, two were health service professionals, two were carers and two came from the NHS Executive.[3]

The interviews

The primary aims of these semi-structured telephone interviews were (a) to gain a broad range of participant perceptions and experiences of the methods used to elicit user views of health care and (b) to explore possible gaps in current research. The interview schedule consisted of eight main topic areas which included among others:

i)   participants' past or present role in eliciting users' view
ii) methods they have used or have been involved in
iii) strengths and weaknesses of these methods
iv) particular groups and/or purposes for which these methods had performed more satisfactorily than others
v)   methods about which we need to know more
vi) what were the perceived gaps in the current research methods that would merit further research

Interviewing started in mid-October 2000 and had been completed by mid-November 2000. Participants were assured that the interview data would be treated as confidential, data would only be accessible to the research team and that the names of individuals and organisations would not be identified. None of the participants objected to the interviews being recorded or the stipulation that the interview material might be utilised for the preparation of scholarly publications. Interviews varied in length, ranging from thirty minutes at the shortest to ninety minutes at longest.

Each interview began with a brief description of the study, its aims and objectives, and the opportunity for the interviewee to ask questions if they so wished. Flexibility in the application of the interview schedule was encouraged to allow for unanticipated views to emerge. The schedule was also amended to suit the particular individual being interviewed or the organisation that they were located in. For example, the focus of the interview for carers was on the methods that they had been involved with and what they liked or disliked about those methods.

The interviews were concluded with contact details being exchanged in order that participants could contact the team if they wished, to discuss the interview itself or any other aspect of the study that they wished further information on. Interviewees were also informed about the plans for feedback and for the presentation of findings resulting from the study.

Analysis

Interviews were taped recorded and then transcribed verbatim. In the original study a thematic approach to data analysis was employed in order to identify emerging themes across all interviews. To aid comprehension and analysis the research team listened to each tape several times as well as reading the associated transcript a number of times. This process was designed to identify anything interesting or significant that the interviewee had said as well as identifying important themes arising within and across the transcripts. Themes were coded according to their content. Emerging themes, some of which were governed by the questions on the interview schedule, were then compared with other transcripts. This process depended upon the content of the themes and not whether respondents agreed or disagreed.

The material being presented here is a secondary analysis of the original research data, an analysis that has been carried out by the author of this chapter not the original researcher, and one that has aimed throughout to be a critical treatment of the themes arising which are pertinent to the subject of this book. The new analysis has involved rearranging the original themes in order to sift out the content of opinions concerning using users of health services in research. Yet, at the same time, it is admitted that some might see this as a contentious exercise since we are now confronting largely decontextualised pieces of narrative that were gathered for a quite different purpose. However, despite these reservations it is a worthwhile exercise as the substance of what these professionals in the academic, health and voluntary sectors have to say do provide a critical window through which to view the actual practice of incorporating the users of health services into research, including its empirical, epistemological and financial bases. The interviewees express real concerns and are acutely aware of the many deficiencies in understanding and practice which are to be found.

Notes

1. This study was undertaken by a group called CHePAS (Consumer Health Psychology at ScHARR).
2. With special thanks to Dr Karen Collins who originally carried out these interviews and provided the initial analysis for the study.
3. Little contextual information is provided about these respondents as some had been concerned that they should not be indirectly identified.

Reference

Blaxter, M. (1995) *'Consumers and Research in the NHS'* London: NHS Executive.

Part Two
Methods

4

Seeking the Views of Consumers Using Quantitative Measures: Patient Experience Surveys

Steven Bruster

Introduction

This chapter looks at the most common method of quantitatively seeking the views of consumers of healthcare – namely surveys. For the purpose of this chapter, 'consumers' are the people who actually use the British National Health Service (NHS) as well as health care systems in other countries, that is the patients. 'Methods' refers specifically to survey methods. The surveys described below are designed to explore the views of consumers and/or patients, or those that can best represent patients – for example their parents or carers.

The chapter looks briefly at the definitions and scope of survey research and some of the key methodological considerations necessary for designing good quality surveys. It is not written as a 'how to design surveys' guide, there are plenty of texts that offer this advice. Rather, it seeks to critically review the current use of surveys and their strength and weaknesses, in accessing the views of consumers. The British NHS Patient Survey Programme conducted in England, will be used as a case study. This is the most comprehensive programme of surveys carried out to assess the views of a patient group about health care, and feeds into annual performance indicators published about NHS Organisations. In particular, two key issues that are rarely given the prominence they deserve are highlighted:

1.   That the research is relevant to the patient population and covers the issues that patients define as important.
2.   That the survey is designed to deliver actionable results. The discussion at the end of this chapter outlines the concerns expressed among the health and social care research community about the variety of tools available that increase the opportunities for poorly trained and uninformed researchers to conduct survey research.

If the aim of the research is to seek the views of patients towards improving the quality of patient care, then there is little real evidence that this approach has been particularly successful. Reasons include that previous research failed to meet the minimal standards of conceptual or methodological rigour (Cleary, 1999; Draper & Hill, 1995), have been unclear in their objectives (Dixon & Carr-Hill, 1989), have been haphazardly administered (Heyden, 1993), use a wide variety of methods (Steele, 1992), have rarely focused on the clinical issues of importance to patients, and have rather covered 'hotel' aspects of healthcare such as food and the hospital environment (Fitzpatrick, 1991; Edgman-Levitan & Cleary, 1996). (See also the views of researchers outlined by Wilson in Chapter 3 which include that research rarely produces 'evidence' that is actionable).

However, there has been increasing recognition that survey research methods are improving (Delbanco, 1995) and that results from well-designed surveys can be useful (Weston D. et al, 1995; Wedderburn-Tate et al, 1995; Stevens L. et al, 1995). Much effort has been directed towards developing rigorous methods for capturing the views of patients that reflect the quality of care, and provide actionable results to health care workers to enable them to improve quality.

The Picker Institute, which has been appointed to be a National Advice Centre for patient surveys, has used carefully developed and tested survey instruments in the USA (Cleary et al, 1993) since 1990 and the UK since 1993 (Bruster et al, 1994) and publishes validation of the survey instruments (Jenkinson et al, 2001).

What is quantitative research?

Quantitative research aims to measure or quantify issues that are already known. It is not, like qualitative research, looking to find or explore new ideas. Quantitative research typically aims to assess frequency and prevalence of a particular behaviour, concept, or other observable practice amongst a population. For example, of all patients at a particular health care organisation having an operation, what percentage is told the risks of the surgery? What percentage of patients visiting the Emergency Department of a hospital is seen within 15 minutes? It *should* be a highly scientific, objective method, concerned with standard approaches and measured by tests of validity and reliability.

Surveys of consumer perspectives are a common part of our everyday lives. For example, at the hotel, on the airline, on the train and in the post-office, surveys are used to examine the experience or satisfaction of consumers. Healthcare providers at hospitals or GP practices increasingly carry out surveys.

Surveys are easy to design, cheap and easy to administer, quick and easy to complete, and quick and easy to analyse. However, carrying out valid, reliable and meaningful research in this area, to drive and support quality improvement, is less easy and does require knowledge of research methods. There is good evidence that well designed survey methods can be useful, not only for measuring the views of patients, but also in contributing to quality improvement (Cleary et al, 1993).

Survey methods in health care

Increasingly, for instance, within the British NHS, surveys are mandatory. By mid-2004 patients from every hospital, every GP practice, every ambulance Trust in England is to have been surveyed as part of a requirement from the British Commission for Health Improvement (CHI).

It is easier now than ever before to conduct survey research. Specialist skills such as survey design can be made easy by the use of new software packages. In addition printing surveys is cheap and can be done in-house, data entry can be carried out quickly and efficiently using scanning technology and data analysis in Windows based packages such as the Statistical Package for the Social Sciences (SPSS) requires no formal knowledge of statistics or survey methods. There are computer hardware and software packages that allow all of the above, a system that allows anyone to design, print, and scan-in and analyse surveys almost at the touch of the button.

As a result, however, work that would have been carried out by researchers with specialist training, knowledge and experience can now be carried out by anyone with access to the necessary tools and equipment. Thus, doctors, nurses, physiotherapists and managers, all experts in their own field, can be observed confidently conducting survey research instead of experts. This is problematic in that it potentially renders results meaningless because these health care professionals often have no expertise at any level of the design and methods for conducting the survey or analysis of the resulting data.

Furthermore, there are other ways of seeking feedback from patients that are becoming more accessible to health care professionals. Traditional methods such as face-to-face or telephone interviewing and self-completion paper surveys, that may have been run by specialist research or market research organisations with great experience, still exist. However, these are now supplemented by a new wave of 'high-tech' providers of surveys where the operators know a great deal about the *technology* of using the various systems such as the internet, automated scanning systems, digital television and implementing consumer feedback into the bedside information systems being installed at many hospitals in the UK and so on, but alarmingly little about the relevant methodological and conceptual issues necessary for design and analysis.

As conducting surveys becomes cheaper, easier and less reliant on specialist skills, so the number of surveys being carried out will continue to grow. Response rates appear to be falling, and poorly designed, irrelevant surveys that are difficult to complete will not help. The bad surveys will impact on the responses to the good ones.

The National Survey Programme in England

There has been increasing interest from central government in using survey methods to seek the views of NHS users, including large national surveys of General Practice in 1999 (Airey et al, 1999) and 2002 (Boreham et al, 2003), Heart Disease in 2000 (Airey et al, 2000) and Cancer in 2001 (Airey et al, 2001). There may be large-scale surveys related to National Service Frameworks in order to measure experience and monitor progress. However the profile of such methods has increased significantly in recent years as such methods are now routinely used to assess the quality of patient care at all NHS Trusts in England.

The Commission for Health Improvement (CHI) currently assesses each NHS Trust (NHS provider such as hospital, primary care, ambulance Trust) in England annually on a range of performance measures. Performance indicators are calculated and star ratings are published each year for each Trust. This information is publicly available, is often featured in local newspapers (particularly for poor performing 'zero star' Trusts) and may have an effect on whether additional moneys are available to the Trust.

Many of the issues of concern to patients, particularly in regard to accessing healthcare (e.g. waiting less than 6 months for an outpatient appointment) and clinical outcomes (e.g. death within 30 days of a heart bypass operation) are included in the performance indicators through the reporting of routinely collected data. However, in addition to such measures, and of equal importance in the performance indicators are patients' views and experiences.

An annual National Patient Survey Programme is currently running in England, and each year NHS Trusts are required to carry out particular specified surveys of their patients. The surveys are based on an approach developed and used by Picker Institute Europe. Information on the development of the inpatient survey is published (Reeves et al, 2002). In the first two years of the programme surveys of inpatients, outpatients, emergency department and primary care have been carried out and included in the performance indicators, with all Trusts to be included in the indicators in future years. Up to June 2003, over 325,000 patients had returned surveys about their healthcare experiences.

As surveys are now part of performance indicators, Trust managers and directors are now very keen to see survey results, to understand what they mean, and to make plans to tackle any resulting issues so as to improve performance ratings in the future. The reliability and validity of such surveys, as used in the Performance Indicators, is key.

Although not all aspects of survey methodology can be covered here in this chapter, the following items are some of the considerations taken into account for the National Survey Programme. These all point towards good quality survey research.

i)   Advice Centre – a national advice centre has been set up to co-ordinate surveys, advise health care organisations and to help with methodology.

ii) Standard methodology – all Trusts have to follow a detailed set of *guidance* so that the survey is carried out identically at all Trusts.

iii) Selecting patients – as the survey results have to be representative of a population (in this case all patient at an NHS Trust), the *sample* has to be well designed. All surveys are based on *random samples* of patient using the service within a particular time period. Specific guidance shows inclusions and exclusions.

iv) Sample size – the sample size is chosen based on estimated *confidence intervals* and the cost-benefit of particular levels of confidence.

v)   *Relevant* – covering the issues of concern to patients.

vi) Surveys are mailed to patients at home- the most efficient way to distribute surveys, but it is also felt that patients may not be completely honest about their experience if they are asked to complete the survey while still at the hospital.

vii) Free – it is free for patients to participate in the survey (FREEPOST envelopes are provided) and there is a FREEPHONE helpline for patients with any queries.

viii) Timely – surveys are ideally mailed to patients soon after a recent healthcare experience. This will allow them to remember what happened and helps to ensure that the survey will normally be important and relevant to them.

ix) Response rates – methods are used to maximise response rates. Two reminders are used for non-responders. The first a letter or postcard and the second a new survey and freepost envelope. In the inpatient surveys, responses after each mailing were typically: 40 per cent after the first mailing, 55 per cent after the first reminder, and 70 per cent after the second reminder. Three weeks is normally left between mailings.

x) Easy to complete – surveys are designed by experienced researchers, and tested using cognitive interviews (SCPR, 1996) and a mailed pilot-test. Some of the measures taken to ensure that surveys are easy to complete have included: avoidance of double-barrelled questions, proverbs, double negatives and the inclusion of 'Don't know' and 'Not applicable' as options. The use of simple words, avoidance of acronyms, abbreviations, jargon, technical terms, ambiguity and leading questions (Oppenhiem, 1992).

xi) Questions are designed to give actionable results.

Two of these issues are rarely given prominence in mainstream survey design. These include that the survey is relevant (covering the correct issues) and that the questions asked lead to actionable results.

Does the survey cover the correct issues? (Relevance)

One of the main considerations for the National Survey Programme, as the NHS aims to become more patient focused, is that quality measures reflect the concerns of patients *as they see them*. This is relevant to all survey research. Too often, managers, clinicians or researchers have designed surveys of patients without any regard as to what the priorities of the patients might be. As noted, this can lead to surveys covering the wrong issues. Research has shown that clinical staff are not good at predicting what is important to patients (Laine et al, 1996).

So, the key starting point for any piece of survey research involving patients is to ensure that the questions that are asked are the correct ones and that therefore, the patients contribute to the design of the survey. Although it may be possible to find out from a number of sources what the key issues for patients might be, for example the media, previous research, complaints letters, speaking with staff, there is no substitute for asking patients themselves to identify the key issues and what is most important to them.

For all of the surveys used as part of the National Survey Programme and all surveys designed by Picker Institute Europe, a significant amount of development has been undertaken with patients. It must be recognised that good quantitative work has to be based on a foundation of good qualitative work and so much of the development work has been based on qualitative work with patients in the form of focus groups or in-depth interviews. Focus groups and in-depth interviews help to explore, with patients, the issues that concern them most about a recent healthcare experience.

Using good qualitative methods it is possible to develop a list of issues that are important to patients (see Chapter 7). However, using such methods does not show which issues are most important to patients or how prevalent these concerns are in the wider population. In order to arrive at a list of the most important issues, two methods are commonly used. Patients can be asked to sort a set of cards which showed particular issues into order from most important to least important (see Chapter 5). Alternatively, or additionally, patients can be asked, as part of a postal survey, to say whether an issue is very important, fairly important, not very important, or not at all important. This gives a list of issues from most important to least important from the patient's perspective to cover in a survey.

Do the questions asked lead to 'actionable results'?

Patient surveys in the NHS are often described as 'patient satisfaction' surveys. A search for references using 'patient satisfaction' as key words will produce a list of many thousands of publications. However, the use of satisfaction measures or general ratings measures has been shown to be problematic (Cohen et al, 1996; Bruster et al, 1994). Examples of this type of question, commonly used in surveys of patients are:

- How satisfied were you with the doctors?
- Overall how would you rate your care?
- How would you rate the waiting time to see the doctor?

The approach developed by Picker Institute Europe and used in the National Survey Programme is to ask a detailed set of questions asking patients to report on 'what happened' to them rather than to rate their satisfaction (Cleary and Edgman Levitan, 1997). There are three principal reasons for preferring this approach:

Overly positive results

Surveys that use general satisfaction ratings of healthcare tend to lead to an overly positive view of the healthcare experience, with typically over 90 per cent of patients rating satisfaction with their care, or rating their care as excellent, very good or good. Examples from an inpatient survey in 1993 carried out by Imperial College (Bruster et al, 1994), showed examples of responses to ratings questions as follows:

- Overall rating of care excellent, very good or good   94 per cent
- Helpfulness of nurses very good, good, or average   99 per cent
- Very or fairly satisfied with room or ward   96 per cent

Of the 24 ratings questions reported, 22 had scores of over 90 per cent. Additionally, written comments from patients, and other evidence such as complaints, suggested an overall rating of care of 94 per cent to be overly optimistic.

When the same patients were asked what happened to them, a different picture emerged, with examples of problem areas being as follows:

- No nurse in charge of care   64 per cent
- Admission cancelled by the hospital   10 per cent
- Not told test results   34 per cent
- No discussion with a doctor about discharge   44 per cent

This shows clear evidence that the reporting questions on 'what happened' are painting a more realistic picture of what patients are really experiencing.

Easily influenced by other factors

Responses by patients to general rating questions are likely to be influenced by other factors (Sixma et al, 1998) for example, their expectations of the NHS, media stories on the NHS, their clinical outcome following a recent health care experience and their health status at the time of completing the survey. In a recent survey carried out by Picker Institute Europe of 28,270 inpatients in England, there were cases that illustrated this point. In this survey, there were 75 questions that asked patients 'what happened' during their stay in hospital. One person had reported on 46 of the 75 questions that problems had occurred. For example, they had reported that:

- They were in a mixed sex ward
- The toilets were not clean
- They didn't get answers to questions
- That doctors talked in front of them as if they weren't there
- That there was no doctor in charge of their care
- That there were rarely or never enough nurses on duty
- That they wanted to be more involved in decisions
- That they were not told test results
- That they were in pain all or most of their time
- That they were discharged too early

However, they rated their care as excellent. On average, those patients that rated their care as excellent reported problems on 9 of the 75 questions they were asked (12%).

Conversely, of the patients that rated their care as poor, problems were reported on as few as 6 of the 75 questions (8%).

The method of asking patients whether a particular event happened or did not happen is much less likely to be influenced by outside factors.

That the results are useful for quality improvement

In order to be useful for quality improvement, results have to be specific and actionable. In themselves, answers from ratings questions are of little use in helping staff to improve patient care. If we take the example from the inpatient survey results above, 94 per cent rated their care as excellent, very good or good. This is of no help in developing action to improve quality; it is neither specific nor actionable.

The detailed reporting of questions asking patients 'what happened' gives staff specific, detailed information on where the problems exist. These can then be tackled and progress measured over time.

What are the advantages of such an approach?

For the National Survey Programme, the methodology leads to a significant number of advantages.

This approach is cost efficient – large numbers of patients can be surveyed relatively cheaply, with little direct involvement from researchers required once the survey instrument is developed.

- Trusts can be instructed to carry out the survey identically
- Data can be quickly collected
- Analysis can be carried out simply and rapidly, so results are based on a recent experience
- Data from different institutions can be combined to produce national results
- Rankings of Trusts can be produced
- Benchmarks showing good results and exceptional performance can be highlighted
- Confidence in the results can be estimated
- Relationships between items can be explored
- Statistical tests can be applied to determine differences between institutions
- Sub-groups can be analysed
- Weightings can be applied to allow adjustment for bias
- Data items can be combined to produce scores for particular themes
- Change over time can be monitored

What are the disadvantages?

A one size fits all approach

This approach assumes that all participating Trusts are the same, and although it could be argued that most of the Trusts do the same sort of thing, there are some exceptions and some of the specialist Trusts (cancer Trusts, women's Trusts) do work slightly differently from others. In some cases the standard sets of questions developed do not apply as well with these Trusts.

Similarly the approach assumes that all patients follow the same sort of process and have the same priorities or concerns. Although many patients do follow similar routes into, through, and out of healthcare, no one patient has the same experience and so the survey may not be relevant to everyone, and may not pick up patient experiences in exceptional circumstances.

Limited scope

A survey is limited in its scope. Although we know that surveys of 4, 8, 12 or 16 pages all result in a similar response rate assuming the survey is relevant (Jenkinson in press), this approach is at its best when only looking at a particular part of a patient's overall experience. For example, an in-patients survey can cover many, although not all, of the important issues for an inpatient. However, it cannot cover aspects of care that happened before a patient was admitted and what has happened afterwards, so such surveys cannot cover the entire experience for any one patient.

Hard to reach groups

This approach does not work well for 'hard to reach groups' or marginalised groups. In particular patients that have difficulty reading and writing English are normally under-represented as they find it difficult to participate. Although great efforts are made to allow as many patients to participate as possible (use of simple language, well tested survey, help available in different languages), these have very limited impact and other methods are probably more appropriate and more successful (see Chapter 10 for further discussion of hard to read groups).

Does not provide all the answers

The results from the surveys often indicate where problems may lie, but because follow-up questions cannot be asked at the time, it is sometimes necessary to carry out further research using qualitative methods or other more detailed surveys to fully understand what the results mean and where quality improvement efforts should be made.

Conclusion

As indicated above, carrying out survey research with patients is easy and cheap, requiring no particular skills. However, high quality, reliable, valid research does require specialised knowledge of all aspects of the survey process, from design and testing through to analysis and reporting. Knowledge of the limitations of the work is essential.

Many examples of good work are published, but there are many surveys carried out that are not published, or were never meant to be published, where the types of issues described here are given little or no consideration. This often leads to surveys being poorly designed, with no clear purpose, using poorly designed questions, of small numbers of patients and with unreliable results. At best this is a waste of resources (financial and staff), and at worst dangerous, whereby decisions about changes in service delivery are based on flawed and unreliable data. The new developments in terms of new survey packages to enable easy design, implementation and analysis of surveys and the new high-tech provision of surveys may lead to an increase in poor quality research.

The rigorous approach used in the National Survey Programme and the well-designed, tested survey does lead to reliable results to be used for performance indicators. More importantly, the results can be used as sound evidence by local staff to help them with quality improvement.

Survey research such as that described here, cannot be carried out in isolation. It requires significant quantitative input during the design and development phase and may need further qualitative work in order to fully understand the results.

Most importantly, with results now being published as part of performance indicators based on strong survey methods, the data has to be used for quality improvement, and change over time has to be seen.

References

Airey, C., Bruster, S., Calderwood, L., Erens, B., Pitson, L., Prior, G. and Richards, N. (2001) *National Survey of NHS Patients: Coronary Heart Disease 1999. National Report: Summary of Findings*, London: NHS Executive.

Airey, C., Becher, H., Erens, B. and Fuller, E. (2001) *National Survey of NHS Patients: Cancer 1999/2000*, London: NHS Executive.

Airey, C., Bruster, S., Erens, B., Lilley, S., Pickering, K. and Pitson, L. (1999) *National Survey of NHS Patients: General Practice 1998*, London: NHS Executive.

Bullen, N. and Reeves, R. (2003) *Acute inpatient Survey, National Overview 2001/2002*, London: Department of Health.

Boreham, R., Airey, C., Erens, B. and Tobin, R. (2002) *National Survey of NHS Patient: General Practice 2002*, London: NHS Executive.

Bruster, S., Jarman, B., Bosanquet, N., Weston, D., Erens, B. and Delbanco, T.L. (1994) National survey of hospital patients, *British Medical Journal*, 309: 1542–9.

Cartwright, A. (1983) *Health Surveys in practice and in potential*, London: King's Fund.

Cleary, P.D., Edgman-Levitan, S., Walker, J., Gerteis, M. and Delbanco, T.L. (1993) Using patient reports to improve medical care: a preliminary report from ten hospitals, *Quality Management in Health Care*, 2(1): 31–38.

Cohen, G.G., Forbes, J. and Garraway, M. (1996) Can different patient satisfaction survey methods yield consistent results? Comparisons of three surveys, *British Medical Journal*, 313: 841–8.

Cleary, P.D. and Edgman-Levitan, S. (1997) Health Care Quality. Incorporating consumer perspectives and *Journal of the American Medical Association*, 278: 1608–12.

Cleary, P.D. (1999) The increasing importance of patient surveys, *British Medical Journal*, 319: 720–721.

Cleary, P.D., Edgman-Levitan, S., Roberts, M., Moloney, T.W., McMullen, W. and Walker, J.D. (1993) Patients evaluate their hospital care: a preliminary report from 10 hospitals, *Quality Management in Health Care*, 2: 31–38.

Delbanco, T.L. (1995) Quality of care through the patient's eyes: satisfaction surveys are just the start of an emerging science, *British Medical Journal*, 313: 832–33.

Dixon, P. and Carr-Hill, R. (1989) The NHS and its customers III. Customer feedback surveys – a review of current practice. York: University of York Centre for Health Economics.

Draper, M. and Hill, S. (1995) The role of patient satisfaction surveys in a National Approach to Hospital Quality management, Australian Government Publishing Service, Canberra.

Edgman-Levitan, S. and Cleary, P.D. (1996) What information do consumers want and need, *Health Affairs*, 15: 42–56.

Fitzpatrick, R. (1991) Surveys of patient satisfaction. I: Important general considerations, *British Medical Journal*, 302: 887–889.

Heyden, V. (1993) Never mind the quality, *Health Service Journal*, 103: 21.

Jenkinson, C., Coulter, A. and Bruster, S. (2002) The Picker Patient Experience Questionnaire: Tests of data quality, validity and reliability using data from in-patient surveys in five countries, *International Journal for Quality in Health Care*, 14(5): 353–358.

Jenkinson, C., Coulter, A., Reeves, R., Bruster, S. and Richards, N. (in press) Properties of the Picker Patient Experience questionnaire in a randomised controlled trial of long and short form survey instruments, *Journal of Public Health Medicine*.

Laine, C., Davidoff, F., Lewis, C.E., Nelson, E.C., Nelson, E., Kessler, R. and Delbanco, T.L. (1996) Important Elements of Outpatient Care: A comparison of Patients and Physicians Opinions, *Annals of Internal Medicine*, 125: 640–645.

Oppenheim, A.N. (1992) Questionnaire Design, Interviewing and Attitude Measurement. Pinter, London.

Rogers, G. and Smith, D. (1999) Reporting comparative results from hospital patient surveys, *International Journal of Quality in Health Care*, 11: 251–259.

Reeves, R., Coulter, A., Jenkinson, C., Cartwright, J., Bruster, S. and Richards, N. (2002) Development and Pilot Testing of questionnaires for use in the acute NHS Trusts inpatient survey programme. Oxford: Picker Institute Europe.

Steele, K. (1992) Patients as experts: consumer appraisal of health services, *Public Money and Management*, 12: 31–37.

SCPR (1996) Using a Cognitive Perspective to Improve Questionnaire Design, *Social & Community Planning Research Survey Methods Centre Newsletter*, 16: 12.

Sixma, H.J. et al (1998) Quality of Health Care from the patients perspective: From Theoretical Concept to a New Measuring Instrument, *Health Expectations*, 12: 82–95.

Straw, P., Bruster, S., Richards, N. and Lilley, S. (2000) Sit up, take notice, *Health Service Journal*, 5704: 24–26.

Stevens, L., Wedderburn-Tate, C. and Bruster, S. (1995) What the patients said, *Health Service Journal*, 5436: 29.

Wedderburn-Tate, C., Bruster, S., Broadley, K., Maxwell, E. and Stevens, L. (1995) What do patients really think? *Health Service Journal*, 5435: 18–20.

Weston, D., Bruster, S., Lorentzon, M. and Bosanquet, N. (1995) The management of quality assurance in nursing, *Journal of Nursing Management*, 3(5): 229–36.

For more information on research carried out by Picker Institute Europe: www.pickereurope.org
For information on the National Survey Programme: www.nhsurveys.org
For information on star ratings: www.chi.nhs.uk/ratings/

5

Using Conjoint Analysis and Willingness to Pay to Determine Consumers' Preferences for Health Care

Alicia O'Cathain and Phil Shackley

Decision makers in health policy and in health care management operate under the constraint of limited resources, where not everything that could potentially benefit consumers can be provided. Therefore, rather than simply elicit consumers' views, they want to identify consumers' strength of preference for different aspects of health care or for different models of service delivery (what they want most), and the trade-offs they are willing to make between different aspects of care (whether they are willing to forgo one thing in order to gain another). That is, they want to determine consumers' perspectives in the context of scarce resources where choices involving sacrifice have to be made. This may present ideological difficulties for those who feel that the National Health Service (NHS) is under resourced and that further provision of resources is a better solution than trading one aspect of a service for another. However, an alternative view is that the provision of more resources for health care will not lead to a situation where all beneficial activities can be provided; there would still be more demands on resources than there are resources to meet those demands and consequently choices would still have to be made.

Preferences and trade-offs are important when individuals make decisions about their own health care. However, in this chapter, we are concerned with consumers making decisions about how services should be provided for themselves and others. Our use of the term 'consumer' refers to patients and service users who have recently received health care, and the general public both as potential recipients of health care and as citizens. Their preferences about service configuration within health care can be determined using a variety of methods, including both quantitative and qualitative techniques, such as simple ranking exercises and citizens' juries (Ryan et al, 2001; Mullen, 1999). (Citizens' Juries are covered in Chapter 6 of this book.) However, only some of these methods can be used to measure *strength* of preference and, in particular, the *trade-offs* people are willing to make between different aspects of services. Two methods commonly used by health economists for these purposes are conjoint analysis (CA) and willingness to pay (WTP). CA is a survey-based technique designed to look at the impact of different characteristics of a service on the overall benefit obtained from that service. It involves presenting individuals with a number of descriptions of services (scenarios), which vary with respect to their characteristics, and asking them to choose their preferred scenario. WTP is a survey-based technique designed to look at how much an individual will sacrifice in monetary terms to obtain a particular service or service characteristic. It involves presenting individuals with descriptions of one or more services and asking them how much they would pay for the service(s). The difficulty of asking consumers to consider payment for services in the context of a health service where care is provided free at the point of delivery is discussed later in the chapter.

Our intention is not to provide a comprehensive review of the literature on CA and WTP, because this has been undertaken elsewhere (Diener et al, 1998; Ryan et al, 2001). Rather our aim is to provide an overview of these techniques specific to the context of consumer health research. In this chapter we describe these techniques in detail, including examples of their use within health research; describe how they have been used to gain consumers' perspectives of health care, including the types of questions they are used to address and the types of services and consumers they have been used with; and then finally describe their strengths and weaknesses in the context of consumer health research.

Conjoint analysis

Conjoint analysis defines a service or intervention in terms of a number of key attributes (e.g. waiting time) and levels (e.g. 3 months or 6 months). The attributes and levels can then be used to define different configurations of the service or intervention for which consumer preferences are elicited. The elicitation of preferences can be done through a ranking, rating or choice-based approach. We will focus mainly on the choice-based approach because it is the most commonly used approach in health care research (Ryan et al, 2001). The choice based approach is typically referred to as a discrete choice experiment or 'discrete choice conjoint analysis' in different publications. (For a more comprehensive description of the method, see Ryan (1999a) or Ryan and Gerard (2003)).

In order to convey the essence of how CA can be applied, we offer a brief description of how the method might work in the context of determining whether the general public in a locality might consider travelling for treatment to shorten their waiting time for an elective operation. A commissioning body, such as a primary care trust, might wish to consider this option for their population, and seek consumer perspectives on it. The following steps would be taken:

STEP 1
Define the attributes of the service. These may be pre-determined by the policy question or identified through literature reviews, expert opinion or directly from consumers. In our example, the two attributes are 'distance to travel' and 'waiting time'.

STEP 2
Assign levels to the attributes. Waiting times might have three levels: one month, three months, and six months, whereas distance might have two levels: local hospital, and hospital in France. Similar methods to those used in identifying attributes can be used to assign appropriate levels.

STEP 3
Construct hypothetical scenarios. These scenarios are defined by the different combinations of attributes and levels. For example one scenario might be 'treatment at a local hospital with a waiting time of six months', while another might be 'treatment in France with a waiting time of three months'.

STEP 4
Reduce the number of scenarios to a manageable level. Unfortunately, even a small number of attributes with relatively few levels can produce a large number of unique scenarios. In such circumstances it may be judged unfeasible to present all of these to each individual, in which case it is common practice to select a smaller subset of scenarios using either mathematical tables or computer packages devised to help with this.

STEP 5
Establish preferences for scenarios. In discrete choice experiments, scenarios are presented to individuals in a series of pairs and individuals asked to indicate their preferred scenario from each pair. For example, one pair-wise comparison might be the choice between having an operation in a local hospital with a 6 month waiting time compared with travelling to France with a three month waiting time. These scenarios can be presented to individuals by postal questionnaire or within a structured interview.

STEP 6
Analyse responses. Regression techniques are used to estimate respondents' relative strength of preference for the different attributes, and trade-offs they are willing to make between different levels of the attributes.

Examples of conjoint analysis studies

Trade-offs between location and waiting time (Ryan et al, 2000)
A CA questionnaire was posted to 1000 members of the general public living on the Isle of Wight to determine whether they would be willing to travel to the mainland for elective surgery, where waiting time would be shorter but travel costs would be greater. Fifty-five per cent of people responded, of whom 78 per cent indicated a willingness to travel. Around a third of respondents were willing to trade between the island and the mainland depending on waiting times and travel costs. A fifth of people were unwilling to travel.

Patients' preferences regarding the process and outcomes of life-saving technology (Ratcliffe & Buxton, 1999)
A CA study was undertaken to assess the relative importance of health outcomes and process attributes, such as waiting time and continuity of contact with medical staff, for liver transplantation services. The attributes were defined using existing literature and 12 interviews with patients. A postal discrete-choice questionnaire was piloted and then sent to 213 patients who had received, rather than were waiting for, transplantation. Fifteen per cent of respondents were not prepared to trade outcomes for process attributes. However, the majority of respondents were willing to trade a reduction in health outcome for an improvement in process characteristics. Respondents were willing to exchange an increase in waiting time to achieve a high level of continuity of care.

Willingness to pay

Willingness to pay, which is also known generically as contingent valuation, is based on the premise that the maximum amount of money an individual is willing to pay for a specific amenity or commodity is an indicator of the value they place on the amenity or commodity. It involves the production of a questionnaire in which the health care programme or intervention is described to respondents who are then asked to state their maximum WTP for the programme or intervention. As with CA, WTP studies can be administered postally or via structured interviews. (For a more comprehensive description of the WTP method, see Donaldson and Shackley (2003)).

The four most commonly used approaches to eliciting WTP values are as follows:

1. *open-ended,* where respondents are asked directly to state their maximum WTP for a service. No prompts or aids are given to respondents.
2. *bidding game,* where individuals are initially presented with a monetary value and asked if they would be willing to pay that amount. Depending upon their response the amount is raised or lowered and the question posed again. This iterative process continues until the maximum value is derived. This method necessitates the use of a structured interview.
3. *payment scale,* where respondents are presented with a range of bids and asked to indicate the value which corresponds to their maximum WTP.
4. *close-ended,* where individuals are presented with a single monetary value and asked whether they would be willing to pay that amount. Different bid amounts are given to different sub-samples, thus allowing the estimation of mean and median WTP. A variation of this approach involves presenting respondents with a follow-up question. Typically, this is either another closed-ended question with a higher or lower amount (depending on the previous response), or an open-ended question.

There is no overall consensus as to which method is to be preferred, with each having advantages and disadvantages. For example, open ended-questions have been criticised by a number of commentators, not least the National Oceanic and Atmospheric Administration (NOAA) Panel which was convened to make recommendations on the conduct of contingent valuation studies for valuing environmental benefits (Arrow et al, 1993). The NOAA panel claimed that open-ended questions provide biased and erratic results. On the other hand, it has been suggested that open-ended questions are valid (Bateman et al, 1994). Similarly, the NOAA panel recommended the use of closed-ended questions on the grounds that, amongst other things, they give conservative estimates of WTP. Yet recent research comparing closed-ended questions with the payment scale approach found that the former gave WTP values which were significantly higher than the values derived from the payment scale (Frew et al, 2003). WTP exercises in health care have tended to use the payment scale and close-ended approaches (Ryan et al, 2001).

Examples of willingness to pay studies

Valuing the benefits of preventing food borne illness (Donaldson et al, 1996)
A random sample of 500 members of the general public in Scotland were sent a self-completion questionnaire in which they were asked to state their WTP for poultry meat which had been irradiated and their WTP for poultry meat which had been treated with a hypothetical device. The question was open-ended and was framed in terms of how much per week respondents were willing to pay over and above their current expenditure on poultry meat. Only those who indicated they would buy irradiated poultry meat were asked their WTP for it. Those who would not buy irradiated meat were asked how much extra they would be willing to pay for meat which had not been irradiated. The authors illustrated how the WTP values and the costs of an irradiation programme could be used to make a policy recommendation on irradiation. Depending on the assumptions used in the estimation, a programme of irradiation was shown to yield a positive net benefit or a positive net cost.

Measuring preferences for maternity care (Donaldson et al, 1998)
WTP was used to value the benefits of different locations of intrapartum care by measuring women's strengths of preference for maternity care and delivery in a midwives' unit relative to care and delivery in a consultant-led labour ward. One hundred and fifty women at low obstetric risk at their booking visit were sent a postal questionnaire, with a response rate of 75 per cent. One third did not express a preference, half expressed a preference for a midwives unit and the remainder preferred a consultant-led service. Although most women preferred the midwives unit, the strength of preference of a small group of low risk women for a labour ward was large.

How have CA and WTP been used to gain consumers' perspectives of health care?

Types of questions addressed

Conjoint analysis has been used mainly to assess preferences for attributes of an established service or treatment, for example what people value most about their out-of-hours primary care (Morgan et al, 2000; Scott et al, 2003), or to consider a new way of delivering a service, for example to determine the trade-offs between location and waiting times in the context of determining whether people would travel for shorter waiting times for elective surgery (Ryan et al, 2000). What has been termed 'social conjoint analysis' has been used to consider the value people place on efficiency and equity in the allocation of liver donors (Ratcliffe, 2000a).

Willingness to pay has been used to determine the value people place on a change to an established service, for example whether people on a waiting list for cataract surgery were willing to pay for a shorter wait (Anderson et al, 1997; Bishai & Lang, 2000), or their preference for a new service or treatment over an established one when health gain is not an issue, for example women's willingness to pay for different models of antenatal care (Donaldson et al, 1998; Ryan et al, 1997). In addition, rather than focusing on a single service, WTP has been used to determine people's priorities for health care expenditure (Olsen & Donaldson, 1998).

One of the strengths of both CA and WTP is their ability to go beyond health outcomes and elicit preferences for processes of care which may be important to consumers. These processes have included continuity of care (Ratcliffe & Buxton, 1999; Ryan, 1996; Ryan et al, 1997), location of services in terms of place or travel time or distance (Jan et al, 2000; Ratcliffe & Buxton, 1999; Ryan, 1996; Ryan et al, 1997; Scott et al, 2003), time spent on the waiting list (Anderson et al, 1997; Jan et al, 2000; Ratcliffe & Buxton, 1999), time spent waiting for a doctor (Jan et al, 2000; Morgan et al, 2000; Ryan, 1996; Scott et al, 2003), amount of information given (Donaldson & Shackley, 1997; Ratcliffe & Buxton, 1999; Ryan, 1996), follow up support (Ratcliffe & Buxton, 1999; Ryan, 1996), ease of parking (Jan et al, 2000), cost (Jan et al, 2000), and doctor's manner (Morgan et al, 2000; Ratcliffe et al, 2002; Ryan, 1996; Scott et al, 2003). These processes can be considered alongside outcomes of care such as treatment complications rates (Jan et al, 2000), success of transplant (Ratcliffe & Buxton, 1999), and symptom relief (Ratcliffe et al, 2002).

The potential importance of valuing processes of care has been demonstrated in a number of studies. For example, people were willing to wait an extra month to have their orthodontic appointment in a local clinic rather than travel to hospital (Ryan & Farrar, 2000), and were willing to take a small reduction of 1 per cent in the chance of a successful liver transplant for an improvement in continuity of care (Ratcliffe & Buxton, 1999). The second of these studies demonstrates that processes of care can be important to consumers even in the context of life-saving services.

Types of services

The techniques have been used to study preferences for a range of services, including emergency care (Leung et al, 2001), secondary care (Anderson et al, 1997; Jan et al, 2000; Ross et al, 2003; Ryan et al, 2000), primary care (Morgan et al, 2000; Ryan et al, 1998; Scott et al, 2003), screening services (Thomas et al, 2000), and complementary therapies (Ratcliffe et al, 2002). One of the most commonly studied areas is women's health, with studies conducted on assisted reproduction (Ryan, 1996), miscarriage (Ryan & Hughes, 1997), antenatal care (Donaldson et al, 1998; Ryan et al, 1997), induction of labour (Taylor & Armour, 2002), and osteoporosis screening (Thomas et al, 2000). Researchers have not shied away from ethically difficult areas, studying life-saving interventions (Ratcliffe & Buxton, 1999) and miscarriage management (Ryan & Hughes, 1997).

Types of consumers

Conjoint analysis has been used with the general public in their capacity as potential service users (Jan et al, 2000; Ryan et al, 2000) and with specific service users such as liver transplant recipients (Ratcliffe & Buxton, 1999) and users of an orthodontic service (Ryan & Farrar, 2000). Service users have also been approached as potential users of a treatment option, for example women attending antenatal clinics were asked about different approaches to induction of labour (Taylor & Armour, 2000).

Willingness to pay has tended to be used more with service users than the general public, for example to determine whether people on a waiting list for cataract surgery were willing to pay for a shorter wait (Anderson et al, 1997), or to determine the views of pregnant women booked at a particular maternity hospital on different ways of offering their maternity care (Donaldson et al, 1998).

Strengths and weaknesses of the methods

Arguably, the main strength of CA and WTP is that they both measure *strength* of preference rather than simply consumer preference. Conjoint analysis identifies the trade-offs individuals are willing to make, while WTP provides a single measure of the value of the benefits of health care. Both techniques reflect the notion that resources are scarce and that choices involving sacrifice have to be made, and they are also firmly rooted in economic theory. Although they are relatively new techniques in health care research, their popularity in health care evaluation is rapidly growing. In addition, a considerable amount of methodological work has been undertaken around their use in other fields such as the environment and transport. Nonetheless there are some questions which researchers, policymakers and consumers may wish to consider prior to commissioning these exercises or interpreting their results.

Have consumers been involved?

An important aspect of CA and WTP is how the service or intervention being valued is presented to respondents. Where possible, in CA it is important to include the attributes which are most relevant to consumers' preferences, whereas in WTP the description should include the aspects of the service or intervention which consumers consider important. It has been recommended that consumers are involved in this process to ensure that the attributes and descriptions are important to them (Wensing & Elwyn, 2002). There is certainly evidence that consumers have been involved in the process to the extent that options for CA have been based on their views. These views are obtained either through a literature review of consumers' views about what is important within a specific service, or through primary qualitative research using group and individual interviews (see Chapter 7). For example, Jan et al (2000) used group interviews to determine attributes that would encourage participants to use one hospital service in preference to another. Four attributes were summarised and used, from the many put forward in the group interviews – travel time, transport/parking, waiting time for elective surgery, and waiting time in accident and emergency. Others have interviewed people experiencing the service under study (Taylor & Armour, 2002; Ratcliffe & Buxton, 1999). Additionally, researchers have recognised that further involvement might be beneficial. For example, Jan et al (2000) wanted to follow up a counter-intuitive finding regarding car parking at hospitals by undertaking group interviews with the general public.

Grounding attributes within the views of consumers, and wanting to explore results with them, is commendable practice. However, there may be benefits from further consumer involvement with these exercises. Consumers could be involved in the design of studies, they could be part of the team which chooses the attributes and levels of attributes in CA exercises, or chooses the bid amounts in WTP exercises, and they could formally assist with interpretation of results. While there may be benefits from moving towards this level of involvement, we must also consider other important stakeholders in the process. Jan et al (2000) added issues relevant to policy makers to the options presented to the general public in their study, such as cost and complications rates, because these issues are important to the funding and planning of hospital services. Others have had their questionnaire reviewed by hospital personnel and clinical colleagues to ensure that it was sensible within the context of services available (Taylor & Armour, 2002; Ratcliffe & Buxton, 1999). The policy relevance of these types of studies may impose choices that consumers do not have much experience with, but nonetheless value, for example complication rates (Jan et al, 2000), or which they may feel uncomfortable about, but are nonetheless important to the larger picture, in particular cost. Thus it is important that consumers are more involved in these types of studies, and that this involvement occurs alongside that of other important stakeholders.

Do consumers find them acceptable?

The acceptability of CA and WTP can be judged by whether consumers respond to the questionnaires, the consistency with which
they complete the questionnaires once they choose to respond,
and the way in which they engage with the exercises. Of course, it
may not be the techniques themselves that are unacceptable, but
sometimes the way in which they are undertaken, for example
very complex scenarios may be constructed in CA studies which
make it difficult for people to engage with these exercises.

Response rates
Obtaining high response rates to questionnaires administered by
post or interview is a challenge for all researchers undertaking
surveys (see Chapter 4), and of extreme importance to ensure
that results are representative of the population sampled. A
variety of factors have been shown to improve survey response
rates, and these include salience of the topic to potential respondents and the number of reminders sent (Edwards et al, 2002).
There is much debate about what a 'good' response rate is, with
Bowling (1997) suggesting 75 per cent. This seems rather high,
but gives a general region for researchers to aim for, while re-
cognising that response rates can be highly dependent on the
population surveyed.

The picture for response rates to CA exercises is mixed. Some
of these exercises, particularly with service users where the topic
of the exercise is of high salience to potential respondents, have
obtained high response rates. Ratcliffe & Buxton (1999) obtained
a response rate of 89 per cent to a postal questionnaire with one
reminder using a covering letter from the hospital consultant.
Ross et al (2003) obtained a response rate of 72 per cent of older
people on a general practice register. However, postal surveys of
the general population concerning preferences for hospital services (Jan et al, 2000), location of services (Ryan et al, 2000), and
attributes of the patient-doctor relationship (Scott & Vick, 1999),
obtained response rates of only 33 per cent, 56 per cent, and 18
per cent respectively. The authors of these studies acknowledge
that they could have increased the response rate through the use
of reminders. It seems sensible, where possible, to follow best
practice for increasing postal response rates when using these

techniques, particularly with the general population. Other things being equal, and if resources permit, surveys administered by interview result in higher response rates than postal administration (McColl et al, 2001).

While none of the published reviews of the WTP literature has reported on response rates (Diener et al, 1998; Klose, 1999; Olsen and Smith, 2001), our reading of the literature suggests that on the whole it seems WTP studies achieve good response rates. For example, 69 per cent of pregnant women (Donaldson et al, 1998), 70 per cent of women attending a scan for screening for osteoporosis (Thomas et al, 2000), and 72 per cent of women in a study of cystic fibrosis carrier screening (Donaldson et al, 1995).

Ease of completion

In CA studies, the majority of respondents typically have little difficulty in answering the questions. For example, in one study 85 per cent of 189 respondents indicated that they had found the exercise 'not difficult' or only 'slightly difficult' (Ratcliffe & Buxton, 1999), while in another study, 80 per cent of 101 respondents stated they found it easy to answer the questions (Vick & Scott, 1998). However, one should not lose sight of the 15–20 per cent of respondents in these two studies who did find the questions difficult. In other studies this percentage has been reported as being as high as 28 per cent and 34 per cent (Ryan & Hughes, 1997; Morgan et al, 2000). Ryan et al (2000) point out that difficulty may arise from choices being inherently difficult to make, or because of the complexity of CA itself, and that this needs further exploration. There is evidence that people have few problems answering WTP questions (Ryan et al, 2001).

The amount of time respondents spend completing a CA questionnaire on average has been found to be somewhere between 12 minutes (Scott et al, 2003) and 16 minutes, although this ranged between 10 and 60 minutes for individuals (Ratcliffe & Buxton, 1999). Thus the response burden seems reasonable on average, although it could be significant for some individuals.

Quality of questionnaire completion

A typical method of testing the internal consistency of CA questionnaires, that is, determining the proportion of respondents who have answered in a logical and consistent manner, is to include a dominant scenario in one of the pairwise choices, the expectation being that consistent respondents will always choose the dominant option. For example, it would be expected that, other things being equal, respondents will prefer a scenario with a shorter waiting time, lower cost, and a lower complication rate. For anyone not choosing this scenario, a case could be made for removing them from further analysis on the grounds that they have not understood what is being asked of them. In practice the percentage of respondents giving illogical answers tends to be small, for example only 2 out of 231 respondents (Jan et al, 2000). However, this percentage can be as large as 7 per cent (Scott et al, 2003) and 9 per cent (Ratcliffe & Buxton, 1999).

A typical method of determining consistency in WTP studies is to ask people to provide an ordinal rank of the options being evaluated and to compare this explicit ranking with the ranking implied from WTP values. Some examples of studies where inconsistencies have been found are Donaldson et al, 1997; Olsen & Donaldson, 1998; Ryan et al, 2001 and Shackley & Donaldson, 2002. One reason put forward to explain the inconsistencies is that some respondents may have been attempting to estimate the cost of the interventions being evaluated rather than the value to them of the interventions (Donaldson et al, 1997; Ryan et al, 2001).

Unwillingness to trade in CA studies

It is important to note that not all responders to CA questionnaires are 'traders', that is, are willing to accept an improvement in one attribute to compensate for deterioration in another. The percentage unwilling to trade can be as low as 0 per cent (Ryan, 1999b) and 16 per cent (Ryan & Hughes, 1997), but as high as 54 per cent (Ryan & Farrar, 2000) and 61 per cent (Bryan et al, 1998). The importance of non-trading is dependent on the context of the research. For example, 15 per cent of people who had undergone a liver transplant were unwilling to trade a change in health outcome for a change in processes of care (Ratcliffe & Buxton, 1999), leaving a significant majority who were willing to do so in the context of a life threatening condition.

The response of some researchers to non-traders has simply been to remove them from their analysis (Ryan & Farrar, 2000), which could mean excluding over half of respondents (Bryan et al, 1998). Researchers recognise that it seems intuitively wrong to remove large numbers of people from the analysis (Ryan & Farrar, 2000) and others have undertaken two analyses, with non-traders included and then excluded, reporting that the results are similar (Ratcliffe & Buxton, 1999). It is important for researchers to report the proportion of people unwilling to trade, and the effect that their removal has on the analysis. It is also important for policy makers to consider non-traders.

Protesters to the concept of WTP

One of the consequences of conducting WTP exercises in publicly-funded health care systems such as the NHS where health care is effectively 'free' at the point of consumption, is that individuals often find it difficult to accept the notion of paying for health care. This tends to manifest itself with a proportion of respondents to WTP exercises protesting at being asked to consider paying for health care at the point of consumption. The protest is typically made by stating a zero WTP and citing such reasons as 'users should not pay' or 'I pay enough taxes already'. Potential ways of minimising this problem include emphasising that the exercise is hypothetical and to find ways of making it as acceptable to respondents as possible. For example, asking people to consider paying via taxation in the United Kingdom or through private insurance premiums in the United States may help. Whatever methods are employed, however, it is unlikely that the problem of protests will be eliminated completely. A typical protest rate in WTP studies in health care is around 10 per cent.

CA versus WTP when studying cost

It has been suggested that a potential solution to the problem of protests to WTP surveys is to derive WTP indirectly in CA studies in which cost is included as an attribute. It has been argued that CA does not meet the resistance met by direct WTP approaches, and that it may even provide more accurate measures of willingness to pay because it eliminates incentives to understate preferences. On the other hand, others argue that WTP is easier for consumers to understand, does not predetermine what people think about in their deliberations and thus allows consumers to incorporate anything into their thinking. Taylor & Armour (2002) have looked at which method may be more acceptable, in the context of women stating preferences for different approaches to induction of labour. The two approaches were placed on the same questionnaire rather than randomly assigned among the women. They found a similarly high response rate to both approaches, with less than 5 per cent of respondents expressing protest votes. However, in one study, cost did not contribute significantly to the model when used as an attribute in CA and the researchers were unable to calculate willingness to pay (Jan et al, 2000). There are methodological concerns when using CA to measure willingness to pay and more research is needed on estimating willingness to pay using CA, with a suggestion that this should be qualitative in nature to determine respondents' cognitive processes (Ratcliffe, 2000b).

Are any consumers disadvantaged?

Any technique which is administered postally is likely to disadvantage people who have difficulty reading (see Chapter 10), making CA and WTP no different from other quantitative techniques such as patient satisfaction surveys (see Chapter 4). Thus attention must be given to people who may not have responded to these exercises, such as people who do not have English as a first language. However, CA and WTP may face the additional difficulty of being inappropriate for use with some 'quiet voices', such as people with learning difficulties and children, because they may be unable to engage with the complexity of the task. There is no evidence that these techniques cannot be used in such groups but it seems likely that there would be problems with this which might result in the exclusion of some voices from participating in processes of decision-making which rely on these techniques. This is discussed further in Chapter 10.

An additional issue with WTP is that it is a function of ability to pay. Indeed, the relationship is often used to test the validity of study results. One consequence of the dependence of WTP on ability to pay is that there is a danger that the preferences of those with higher incomes are given greater weight than those with lower incomes, leading to a situation where resources are allocated on the basis of ability to pay. A possible solution to this problem is to weight responses by income band (see Donaldson (1999) for a detailed discussion of this issue).

Do we understand how consumers engage with these exercises?

While it seems that consumers, by and large, are willing to engage in CA and WTP surveys, we do not fully understand the thought processes of individuals when they complete these exercises. Verbal protocol analysis, where people talk through their thought processes as they complete a willingness to pay exercise, has been used in environmental WTP research and shown that people were not completing the exercise as intended (Schkade & Payne, 1994). Concern has been expressed that consumers may not have preferences which can simply be measured, that they process information in different ways which are dependent on how that information is presented to them, and that they may take cognitive shortcuts to simplify the task in hand (Lloyd, 2003). There is a growing need to understand the reasons why people hold certain preferences, and whether they are completing the questionnaires in the ways intended by the researchers. It has been suggested that qualitative research on the cognitive strategies adopted when completing these quantitative tools needs to be undertaken (Ryan et al, 2001).

Do consumers do what they say they will do?

The values derived from CA and WTP studies are, by their very nature, hypothetical. An obvious question to ask is do the hypothetical values reflect the values people would reveal in reality, i.e. are the values externally valid? A review of the literature of studies outside health care found that, compared with revealed preference methods, contingent valuation WTP estimates tend to be lower (Carson et al, 1996). One study in the health literature has shown that a revealed preference and contingent valuation method arrive at similar valuations (Kennedy, 2002), whilst others have shown the opposite to the review (Clarke, 1997), with one also making the claim that it may still be possible to correct for the overestimation (Blumenschein et al, 2001). Further research is clearly necessary, although such research is difficult in the publicly-financed NHS. It may be fruitful to explore this in the context of private health care and complementary and alternative therapies.

Who should participate?

Both techniques can be undertaken with the general public and service users. Shackley & Ryan (1995) argue that the general public would most appropriately participate in an exercise about the availability of services in their community, whereas service users would most appropriately participate in an exercise about the attributes of the service they use. However, it is not always easy to decide who is the most appropriate recipient of the questionnaire. Ratcliffe & Buxton (1999) sent their CA questionnaire to people who had undergone liver transplant in the previous ten years. These people had survived the transplant and the authors acknowledge that the results may have been different had the survey been sent to patients *awaiting* treatment. They had concerns that prospective patients might have difficulty determining the importance of attributes they had not experienced, whereas experienced users would express informed preferences. Additionally, they were concerned about generating anxiety in this patient group.

There are also issues about who should participate in WTP exercises. For example, when using WTP in the context of a randomised trial, it has been argued that there are problems with surveying actual trial participants, and that instead preferences should be elicited from a group of patients with the same characteristics as trial patients, but who are not participating in the trial themselves (Donaldson et al, 1995; Donaldson et al, 1997; Shackley & Donaldson, 2000).

What are the methodological challenges?

We do not intend to go into detail about the methodological and analytical concerns surrounding these techniques (Klose, 1999). Generic researchers working in universities, health care organisations such as primary care trusts, or for consumer groups, will need to seek the specialist skills of health economists to apply these techniques, and health economists are well aware of their limitations. However, it is important for everyone to understand the implications of these limitations when interpreting the results of these exercises. The greatest methodological concern for both of these techniques is that changes in the way these exercises are presented to consumers may affect the results (Slothuus et al, 2000). For example, CA involves the reduction of a large number of unique scenarios, often hundreds, to a 'manageable' number such as 18, for presentation to consumers. A different selection of scenarios, and different pairings of these scenarios, may yield different results. Health economists are in the process of establishing the effect of ordering of comparator scenarios, ordering of attributes within scenarios, the choice of comparator, and the number of levels, on preferences. Similarly, WTP may suffer from starting point bias, where the results are sensitive to the starting point in the bidding technique, and range bias in the selection of values presented to respondents in payment methods.

Conclusions

Policy makers and managers make decisions about health care in the context of limited resources. Changes in the way services are delivered may involve sacrifice, for example increasing the provision of local services may be at the expense of increasing waiting time for that service. Both conjoint analysis and willingness to pay are useful techniques for determining the consumer perspective on the value they place on different service characteristics and configurations so that decisions made at a primary care organisation level, say, can incorporate these values. Like all methods, they have their strengths and their weaknesses. Their strengths lie in their ability to measure consumers' *strength* of preference and the trade-offs they are willing to make between different aspects of health care, and the fact that consumers are given the opportunity to express their preferences on the *processes* as well as outcomes of health care. Their weaknesses lie in their acceptability to consumers in that some people find conjoint analysis exercises difficult to answer, and some people register protest votes in willing to pay exercises because they are not willing to engage in even theoretical exercises around paying for a publicly funded service. Both techniques may not be suitable for use with some members of the general public or some patient groups such as people with learning difficulties. Further, they both face methodological difficulties which experts in their use fully recognise (Ryan, 1999; Donaldson et al, 1998) and are actively engaged in addressing. We feel that two issues need particular attention. First, we need to know more about the effect, on the results obtained, of the way in which these techniques are presented to consumers. This is likely to involve quantitative testing of the effect of varying presentations of exercises to consumers. Second, we need to know more about how people construct preferences and make decisions as they complete these exercises and the extent to which the strategies they employ are similar or different to those intended by health economists. This is likely to involve a qualitative approach, with psychologists making close study of the thought processes employed by consumers as they complete these exercises (Lloyd, 2003). Thus both quantitative and qualitative research should be undertaken to help us to understand and refine these methods, alongside their continued use to determine consumer preferences in health care.

References

Anderson, G., Black, C. and Dunn, E. et al (1997) Willingness to pay to shorten waiting time for cataract surgery, *Health Affairs*, 16: 181–190.

Arrow, K., Solow, R. and Portney, P.R. et al (1993) Report of the NOAA panel of contingent valuation, *Federal Register*, 58: 4601–14.

Bateman, I., Willis, K. and Garrod, G. (1994) Consistency between contingent valuation estimates: a comparison of two studies of UK national parks, *Regional Studies*, 28, 457–474.

Bishai, D.M. and Lang, H.C. (2000) The willingness to pay for wait reduction: the disutility of queues for cataract surgery in Canada, Denmark, and Spain, *Journal of Health Economics*, 19: 219–230.

Blumenschein, K., Johannesson, M., Yokoyama, K.K. and Freeman, P.R. (2001) Hypothetical versus real willingness to pay in the health sector: results from a field experiment, *Journal of Health Economics*, 20: 441–457.

Bowling, A. (1997) Research Methods in Health. Investigating health and health services. Open University Press.

Bryan, S., Buxton, M., Sheldon, R. and Grant, A. (1998) Magnetic resonance imaging for the investigation of knee injuries: an investigation of preferences, *Health Economics*, 7: 595–603.

Carson, R.T., Flores, N.E., Martin, K.M. and Wright, J.L. (1996) Contingent valuation and revealed preference methodologies: comparing the estimates for quasi-public goods, *Land Economics*, 72: 80–99.

Clarke, P.M. (1997) *Valuing the benefits of health care in monetary terms with particular reference to mammographic screening*, PhD Thesis, Australian National University, Canberra.

Diener, A., O'Brien, B. and Gafni, A. (1998) Health care contingent valuation studies: a review and classification of the literature, *Health Economics*, 7:313–326.

Donaldson, C. (1999) Valuing the benefits of publicly-provided health care: does 'ability to pay' preclude the use of 'willingness to pay'? *Social Science and Medicine*, 49(4), 551–563.

Donaldson, C., Hundley, V. and Mapp, T. (1998) Willingness to pay: a method for measuring preferences for maternity care? *Birth*, 25: 32–39.

Donaldson, C., Mapp, T. Ryan, M. and Curtin, K. (1996) Estimating the economic benefits of avoiding food-borne risk: is 'willingness to pay' feasible? *Epidemiology and Infection*, 116, 285–294.

Donaldson, C. and Shackley, P. (1997) Does 'process utility' exist? A case study of willingness to pay for laproscopic cholescystectomy, *Social Science & Medicine*, 44: 699–707.

Donaldson, C. and Shackley, P. (2003) Willingness to pay for health care. In Scott, A., Maynard, A. and Elliott, R. (eds) *Advances in Health Economics*, pp. 1–24. Wiley, Chichester.

Donaldson, C., Shackley, P., Abdalla, M. and Miedzybrodzka, Z. (1995) Willingness to pay for antenatal carrier screening for cystic fibrosis. *Health Economics*, 4: 439–452.

Donaldson, C., Thomas, R. and Torgerson, D.J. (1997) Validity of open-ended and payment scale approaches to eliciting willingness to pay. *Applied Economics*, 29: 79–84.

Edwards, P., Roberts, I. and Clarke, M. et al (2002) Increasing response rates to postal questionnaires: systematic review, *BMJ*, 324: 1183–5.

Frew, E.J., Whynes, D.K. and Wolstenholme, J.L. (2003) Eliciting willingness to pay: comparing closed-ended with open-ended and payment scale formats, *Medical Decision Making*, 23, 150–159.

Jan, S., Mooney, G., Ryan, M., Bruggemann, K. and Alexander, K. (2000) The use of conjoint analysis to elicit community preferences in public health research: a case study of hospital services in South Australia, *Australian and New Zealand Journal of Public Health*, 24 (1): 64–70.

Kennedy, C. (2002) Revealed preference compared to contingent valuation: radon-induced lung cancer prevention, *Health Economics*, 11, 585–598.

Klose, T. (1999) The contingent valuation method in health care, *Health Policy*, 47: 97–123.

Leung, G.M., Chan, S.S., Chau, P.Y. and Chua, S.C. (2001) Using conjoint analysis to assess patient's preferences when visiting emergency departments in Hong Kong, *Academic Emergency Medicine*, 8(9): 894–8.

Lloyd, A.J. (2003) Threats to the estimation of benefit: are preference elicitation methods accurate? *Health Economics*, 12: 393–402.

McColl, E., Jacoby, A. and Thomas, L. et al (2001) Design and use of questionnaires: a review of best practice applicable to surveys of health service staff and patients, *Health Technology Assessment*, 5(31).

Morgan, A., Shackley, P., Pickin, M. and Brazier, J. (2000) Quantifying patient preferences for out-of-hours primary care, *Journal of Health Services Research and Policy*, 5: 214–218.

Mullen, P.M. (1999) Public involvement in health care priority setting: an overview of methods for eliciting values, *Health Expectations*, 2:222–34.

Olsen, J.A. and Donaldson, C. (1998) Helicopters, hearts and hips: using willingness to pay to set priorities for public sector health care programmes, *Social Science & Medicine*, 46: 1–12.

Olsen, J.A. and Smith, R.D. (2001) Theory versus practice: a review of 'willingness-to-pay' in health and health care, *Health Economics*, 10, 39–52.

Propper, C. (1991) Contingent valuation of time spent on NHS waiting lists, *Econ J*, 100:193–9.

Ratcliffe, J. (2000a) Public preferences for the allocation of donor liver grafts for transplantation, *Health Economics*, 9: 137–148.

Ratcliffe, J. (2000b) The use of conjoint analysis to elicit willingness to pay values, *International Journal of Technology Assessment in Health Care*, 16: 270–290.

Ratcliffe, J. and Buxton, M. (1999) Patients' preferences regarding the process and outcomes of life-saving technology, *International Journal of Technology Assessment in Health Care*, 15;2: 340–351.

Ratcliffe, J., Van Haselen, R., Buxton, M., Hardy, K., Colehan, J. and Partridge, M. (2002) Assessing patients' preferences for characteristics associated with homeopathic and conventional treatment of asthma: a conjoint analysis study, *Thorax*, 57: 503–8.

Ross, M.A., Avery, A.J. and Foss, A.J. (2003) Views of older people on cataract surgery options: an assessment of preferences by conjoint analysis, *Quality and Safety in Health Care*, 12: 13–17.

Ryan, M. (1996) Using willingness to pay to assess the benefits of assisted reproductive techniques, *Health Economics*, 5: 543–558.

Ryan, M. (1999a) A role for conjoint analysis in technology assessment in health care, *International Journal of Technology Assessment in Health Care*, 15: 443–57.

Ryan, M. (1999b) Using conjoint analysis to take account of patient preferences and go beyond health outcomes: an application to in vitro fertilisation, *Social Science and Medicine*, 48: 535–546.

Ryan, M. and Farrar, S. (2000) Using conjoint analysis to elicit preferences for health care, *BMJ*, 320: 1530–3.

Ryan, M. and Gerard, K. (2003) Using discrete choice experiments in economics moving forward. In Scott, A., Maynard, A. and Elliott, R. (eds), *Advances in Health Economics*, pp. 25–40. Wiley, Chichester.

Ryan, M. and Hughes, J. (1997) Using conjoint analysis to assess women's preferences for miscarriage management, *Health Economics*, 6: 261–73.

Ryan, M., McIntosh, E., Dean, T. and Old, P. (2000) Trade-offs between location and waiting times in the provision of health care: the case of elective surgery on the Isle of Wight, *Journal of Public Health Medicine*, 22: 202–10.

Ryan, M., McIntosh, E. and Shackley, P. (1998) Using conjoint analysis to assess consumer preferences in primary care: an application to the patient health card, *Health Expectations*, 1: 117–29.

Ryan, M., Ratcliffe, J. and Tucker, J. (1997) Using willingness to pay to value alternative models of antenatal care, *Social Science & Medicine*, 44: 371–380.

Ryan, M., Scott, D.A. and Reeves, C. et al. (2001) Eliciting public preferences for healthcare: a systematic review of techniques, *Health Technology Assessment*, 5(5).

Schkade, D.A. and Payne, J.W. (1994) How people respond to contingent valuation questions: a verbal protocol analysis of willingness to pay for an environmental regulation, *J Environ Econ Manage*, 26: 88–109.

Scott, A., Watson, S.M. and Ross, S. (2003) Eliciting preferences of the community for out of ours care provided by general practitioners: a stated preference discrete choice experiment, *Social Science & Medicine*, 56: 803–14.

Scott, A. and Vick, S. (1999) An application of principle-agent theory to the doctor-patient relationship, *Scott J Polit Econ*, 46: 111–34.

Shackley, P. and Donaldson, C. (2000) Willingness to pay for publicly-financed health care: how should we use the numbers? *Applied Economics*, 32(15), 2015–2021.

Shackley, P. and Donaldson, C. (2002) Should we use willingness to pay to elicit community preferences for health care? New evidence from using a 'marginal' approach, *Journal of Health Economics*, 21, 971–991.

Shackley, P. and Ryan, M. (1995) Involving consumers in health care decision making, *Health Care Anal*, 3: 196–204.

Slothuus, U., Larsen, M.L. and Junker, P. (2000) Willingness to pay for arthritis symptom alleviation. Comparison of closed-ended questions with and without follow-up, *International Journal of Health Technology Assessment in Health Care*, 16: 60–72.

Taylor, S. and Armour, C. (2000) Measurement of consumer preference for treatments to induce labour: a willingness to pay approach, *Health Expectations*, 3: 203–216.

Taylor, S. and Armour, C. (2002) Acceptability of willingness to pay techniques to consumers, *Health Expectations*, 5: 341–356.

Thomas, R., Donaldson, C. and Torgerson, D. (2000) Who answers 'willingness to pay' questions? *Journal of Health Services Research and Policy*, 5: 7–11.

Vick, S. and Scott, A. (1998) Agency in health care. Examining patients' preferences for attributes, *J Health Econ*, 17: 587–605.

Wensing, M. and Elwyn, G. (2002) Research on patients' views in the evaluation and improvement of quality of care, *Quality and Safety in Health Care*, 11: 153–157.

6

Citizens' Juries and the Deliberative Family

Clare Delap

Introduction

Since first being piloted in the UK in 1997 citizens juries and other deliberative methods have become firmly established as a mechanism for involving the public in health care decision-making. A great deal has been learned about the appropriateness of these methods and about the circumstances in which they are most likely to be successful. However, it is harder to say how juries and other deliberative processes have added value or whether they have had an impact. This chapter provides an overview of the role of deliberative methods and has three main aims: Firstly, to look at the reasons for using deliberative methods to involve the public in health care decisions. Secondly, to examine the features of deliberative approaches; and thirdly, to outline lessons from the UK experience about appropriate use with a view to identifying ways in which this method might be used in other countries.

To conclude, I identify and discuss the gaps in existing knowledge of deliberative public involvement and the barriers to creating a more participative culture within the British National

Health Service (NHS) and by implicating other health services across the world.

There are many voices which need to be heard when health policy is made. Individual users of healthcare, those who care for them, and healthcare professionals must be consulted about the services they encounter. However, it has been argued that having a NHS belonging to all members of society demands that a wider *citizen* perspective also be accessed. This is a view-point which takes into account conflicting needs of different groups and is also able to take a longer-term perspective on policy making. The citizens' jury and its application in the UK in the 1990s represents one attempt to bring a citizens' view into health policy making. This chapter also examines to what extent it has been successful.

A citizens' jury brings together a small group of randomly selected individuals or 'citizens' to discuss a matter of public policy over a number of days. During this time they interview 'witnesses' and discuss the issues. At the end of the process they are expected to reach a conclusion and present their findings. The intention is for their findings to make a contribution to public policy.

The use of citizens' juries in the UK

There have been over 300 citizens' juries held in the UK over the last six years on topics ranging from health care priorities to taste and decency on television.[1] Mostly they have been sponsored by public sector agencies such as health and local authorities and central public agencies but some sponsored by industry, particularly the pharmaceutical industry.

The concept of inviting a small group of citizens to become involved in a matter of public concern clearly struck a cord within the health policy field. At this time the legitimacy of unelected health authorities, and the democratic deficit in local government was causing particular concern (Cooper et al, 1995). In particular, the way that decisions were being taken about allocating health care resources was under increasing scrutiny. It was no coincidence that one of the first agencies to pilot citizens' juries was Cambridge and Huntingdon Health Authority where the 'Child B' case had caused such uproar.[2]

Support from the new British Labour administration was also key to the initial take-up of citizens' juries. The Government promoted new approaches to public participation as a way of reinvigorating interest in local government and counteracting public concern about a series of health policy decisions (Lowndes et al, 1998).[3] This strong interest from the centre, combined with mounting criticisms around the accountability of much of the health service led to a wave of experimentation in new forms of involvement and to the establishment of citizens' juries and other deliberative methods as part of the 'toolkit' of public involvement (Stewart, 1996).

However, in some areas at least, citizens' juries appeared to suffer a quick burnout. Despite initial enthusiasm there have been very few run in the health field in the last few years. There are a number of possible explanations for this.

Firstly, that much too soon was claimed for deliberative methods before their real potential was fully examined. Citizens' juries are time consuming and expensive, and decision-making bodies are right not to use them lightly. It is also true that the policy agenda has moved on. The interest now lies in creating a new set of institutions, rather than in a series of public involvement initiatives from the 1990s.[4] Lastly it has been argued that the uncontrollable outcomes of citizens' juries, their open and public nature, represents a danger to policy makers – it is safer to put funding into methods of research where those in power have more control over the process (Wakeford, 2002; Parkinson, 2003).

Deliberative approaches are extremely relevant to the NHS today. I go on to outline the elements of deliberation and to describe the attempts to realise them through citizens' juries and other models.

Citizenship and deliberation

The citizens' jury approach was developed from a critique of *who* is involved in decision making about health and issues of public policy, and *how* people take part in those decisions. It was argued that questions of public concern, such as the prioritising of healthcare resources, demand a *citizen* perspective. Lenaghan suggested that while individual users of healthcare are concerned with their own immediate needs as patients:

> *'Citizens have a broader and longer-term interest in the health service, as voters, taxpayers and members of the community: they are interested in what happens not only to themselves, but also to their families, neighbours and fellow citizens, both now and in the future'. (Lenaghan, 1999)*

As well as improving the way decisions are made including the citizen perspective will help re-democratise and re-invigorate democratic activity (Stewart et al, 1997). It also has the potential to create a more active citizenship in which a wider body of people are involved in discussions on a collective basis (Rogers, 2003).

But how to access a citizen perspective? It was clear that conventional methods from opinion surveys to public meetings were inadequate because they did not give people the time and the space to understand the complex issues at hand and to reach decisions based on the collective good. Conventional research also placed the subject in a passive role as an object of study rather than as an active contributor (Barnes, 1999).

A deliberative approach offers an alternative way of involving local people in matters which concern them. Very briefly, deliberative democracy is concerned with a process of transformation. Rather than assuming that values are fixed and that democracy is about exchanging individual preferences, it sees democracy as a forum which can create common values through public debate (Smith & Wales, 2000; Parkinson, 2003; Renn & Webler, 1995). It is a concept based on *dialogue* between citizens and between citizens and those in positions of power. In practice a deliberative approach demands mechanisms which enable *inclusive, reasoned debate* between *equals* (Smith and Wales, ibid).

Inclusivity is an important but contested concept for deliberative democracy. A citizens' jury is randomly selected and (within certain boundaries) anyone can be invited to attend one (Crosby, 1995). For some commentators inclusivity demands the 'presence' of those not normally heard (see Barnes, 1999, see also Chapter 10). Reasoned debate involves discussion with other citizens and the chance that participants can change their views. For Dryzeck a group is deliberatively rational when its 'interactions are egalitarian, uncoerced, competent and free from delusion, deception, power and strategy' (quoted Smith and Wales, 2000). Thus the independence of such mechanisms is clearly critical, that they are constructed in such a way to free them from political manipulation. In practice there are problems with these concepts as we shall see below but the citizens jury and related approaches are all concerned with creating forums for common, inclusive debate in which citizens play an active part.

The citizens' jury

The citizens' jury adopted in the UK is based on German Planning Cells and American Citizens' juries and has many similarities to approaches in other parts of Europe (Crosby, 1995; Dienel & Renn, 1995; Font, 2001).

The basic principle of a citizens' jury is to invite a group of randomly selected citizens to consider a matter of policy. Participants are offered time to discuss their ideas and information to help them reach conclusions. 12–16 local people are selected to match a rough cross-section of the local community. Various recruitment methods can be used, one being to write to a random sample from the Electoral Register advising them of the jury process and inviting their participation. From these responses, the actual jury is recruited. Many practitioners prefer to use professional recruiters to approach individuals and fulfil a quota that matches a sample of the local population (Clarke et al, 2001). The jurors are not 'representative' in any demographic sense, but they are expected to include people from a range of local backgrounds. In order to enable as full a range of people as possible to attend incentives such as honorarium payment, help with travel to and from the jury venue and jury hearings at convenient times are offered to participants (Coote & Lenaghan, 1997).

A jury will sit for between two and a half days and four and a half days, depending upon the complexity of the question and subject matter.[5] Jurors will be asked to address a question or questions on an important matter of policy or planning. Typically, there will be two moderators working with the jury to assist them in exploring and examining the question from all dimensions. The jurors will work in plenary sessions, small groups, pairs and individually to ensure that everyone has the opportunity to fully contribute to the process.

Jurors are fully briefed, receive all evidence and have the opportunity to cross-examine witnesses. They will discuss the issues fully, with witnesses and amongst themselves. They have an opportunity to ask for further information and to call their own witnesses. At the end of the event jurors draw together their conclusions and recommendations and present them to the commissioning body. The jury proceedings are compiled in a report to which the commissioning body is expected to respond.

Citizens' juries have a number of specific key features:

- Participants are selected or recruited rather than accepting an open invitation to a public meeting
- Information is offered to participants who are given the opportunity to scrutinise different viewpoints and options
- Participants are given time to reflect on the questions at hand
- The jurors are expected to develop a shared view of the question/s they have been asked to address. The momentum of the process, including the style of moderation and the way the agenda is structured, reflects this objective.

Juries also represent a policy-oriented process: they have been designed to feed into the actual decisions being taken by public bodies. Most citizens' juries are attempting to answer a particular 'charge' defined by a public body such as how best to improve palliative health care in the area (Coote and Lenaghan, 1998). The agenda for the jury can be structured in a way which is independent and open to citizens' views but which is focused on the concerns of policy makers (McIver, 1998). This does however, lay the process open to complaints of manipulation by those in power (see below).

Related approaches

There are many other deliberative approaches currently being used in the UK. They all share some of the features of the citizens' jury and a few are listed below.

Approach type	Description	Examples
Re-convening groups	A focus group that meets more than once to further discuss information provided	Department for the Environment, Food and Rural Affairs consultation on sustainable development
Deliberative Opinion Polls	Measuring opinion before and after information has been provided, involve 200–600 people	Granada Polls run by the National Centre. See Fishkin, 1997
Consensus Conferences	15–20 people who meet 3 or 4 times to discuss an issue and question experts	UK Centre for Economic and Environmental Development Consensus Conference on Radioactive Waste, 2000
Planning for Real	A hands on visual means of involving local people in planning	Neighbourhoods Initiative Forum have trademarked the name, been run since the 1970s.
Workshops	A variety of formats but normally a day event involving between 15–30 people	National Consumer Council workshops looking at the views of low income consumers on food and farming, 2002
Visioning exercises such as Future Search	A Future Search Conference brings together stakeholders (around 60) and involves them in structured meetings to agree and commit on a shared approach	New Economics Forum and the Office for Public Management have run several of these

Many other institutions and approaches may well be described as 'deliberative'. For instance some of the structures set up within local and health authorities to involve the public or specific users share some, if not all, deliberative features.[6] There is a danger of becoming too pre-occupied in the names of tools rather than designing deliberative processes to suit a purpose (see Cabinet Office, 2002). It is more useful therefore to speak in terms of some key deliberative elements.

Elements of deliberation

To various extents deliberative approaches can be distinguished from conventional forms of research because they include:

> *Deliberation or discussion: rather than asking for immediate opinions, all these approaches ask participants to discuss issues with fellow citizens before deciding their views. Thus the results can be seen to represent what the public would say if they were given the chance to discuss issues (Fishkin, 1995).*

> *Time: to an extent it is expected that complex issues need a degree of time for reflection (Coote & Lenaghan, 1997).*

> *Information: to help citizens come to their conclusions they are helped to varying degrees by neutral expert information.*

There are of course huge differences between the approaches, which depend on different roles appointed to the participant. Deliberative approaches differ in a number of ways:

- *The level of information received by participants:* Harrison and Mort found great differences between the amounts of information received in different discursive forums. (Harrison and Mort, 1999, see also Combe et al, 1999 for further discussion)
- *The amount of time participants are given to reflect and the amount of discussion undertaken:* while of course this depends on the question being examined, some deliberative approaches take a few hours while others take a few days.
- *The extent to which they are expected to make a decision:* Some groups are expected to reach some kind of collective conclusion (like a jury) whereas others are not (as in a deliberative opinion poll, or a planning for real exercise).
- *How participants are recruited:* some use similar methods to citizens' juries, others adopt a more open invitation approach such as many community events.

Deciding what kind of approach to use is partly a matter of practical choice. There now exist a number of useful guides to help those in public bodies choose from the 'toolkit' of public participation (see for instance Cabinet Office, 2002). However, for many proponents of deliberative democracy, the form that participation takes depends on who participants are and whether the public being constructed is a passive recipient or an active participant in the exercise (Mort and Kashefi, 2001). I will now go on to look at the lessons from the attempt to create arenas for active participation, through citizens' juries.

Discussion: citizens' juries as deliberative democracy?

The initial wave of citizens' juries prompted a fair amount of discussion of the process (Coote & Lenaghan, 1997; Davies et al, 1998), and some evaluations of individual experiences (McIver, 1998; Barnes, 1999; Dunkerly & Glasner, 1998). Since then some useful work has been done on developing generic evaluation tools to establish whether participation has 'worked' (Marsh et al, 2001; IDEA, 2002). But there have been few attempts to compare the experiences of different juries, or to compare the different elements of deliberative approaches (Barnes, 1999; Combe et al, 1999). What conclusions can we then draw about the successes of citizens' juries?

It is argued above how citizens' juries are a practical application of the deliberative goal to create *independent forums* for *inclusive, reasoned debate* among *equals*. Citizens' juries have, to a certain extent, been successful in creating such forums, but commentators have also been extremely critical of their attempts to realise some of the deliberative goals. Their application has raised many questions for those wishing to create more participative decision-making.

Inclusivity

As in a legal jury a citizens' jury is inclusive in principle because any member of the public could take part. The question remains however, how far this has enabled the voices of previously unheard citizens to take part. There have been a few attempts to look at who agrees to take part in juries and these studies have concluded that, generally, those who have taken part are not necessarily the politically active and that they have come from a wide range of backgrounds (Coote & Lenaghan, 1997; McIver, 1998).

However, whether more marginalised voices can be heard in such forums is less certain. Barnes warns that while prioritising a citizen perspective may bring in new voices, there is also a danger that some disadvantaged groups, such as user groups, may not be included in this non-expert citizen role (1999, p. 67). It is important that the entire range of voices must be heard, and to recognise that different types of participant require different approaches (see Chapter 10 which discusses the issues related to marginalised groups).

Reasoned debate amongst equals

The application of citizens juries and other deliberative approaches have led time and again to the conclusion that, given the opportunity, members of the public show competence and confidence in discussing and reaching conclusions about complex matters of policy. On a range of issues those who have taken part in juries have demonstrated concern for one another, subject 'witnesses' to scrutiny, and often rejected options provided for them to produce their own answers to questions (Smith and Wales, 2000; Coote & Lenaghan, 1997; Davies et al, 1998; see also Fishkin, 1997 for comparable experiences on a larger scale).

The immediate reactions of those involved has also been extremely encouraging – almost all the studies demonstrate a great willingness to take part and a positive attitude to the experience – participants report that they have learned a lot from the process, that it has contributed to their own sense of belonging to a community and often to their own sense of worth (McIver, 1998; Clarke et al, 2000). Those in positions of authority who have witnessed juries have, to a large extent, been extremely impressed by the ability demonstrated (Barnes, 1999).

However whether these effects last is much less certain. Any evaluations carried out have been unlikely to re-visit individual jurors. As forums juries have been able to promote a reasoned and considered approach and have demonstrated the possibility that individuals will work together to create a citizens perspective. However, the claims about longer effects on citizenship are much harder to verify.

Legitimacy

Two of the biggest concerns that are raised about deliberative forums like citizens' juries are their cost, and the small numbers of people involved compared to conventional forms of research. In a world driven by opinion polling, how can health care managers justify spending such large sums on an event involving so few people?[7] How can a citizens' jury be seen as a legitimate public voice when so few members of the public are directly involved? The legitimacy of a jury, as in a legal jury, rests on the acceptance that the process has been conducted in a fair and competent manner. As Wakeford puts it: 'once a small sample of a population have heard the evidence, their subsequent deliberations can fairly represent, the conscience and intelligence of the community' (2002, p. 1). This legitimacy can be established in three ways: through the *perceived independence of the process*, through *publicity*, that the wider community knows about the event and feels in some way connected to it, and through some *tangible proof* of its *effectiveness*.

Independence

It is critical that a process which purports to be democratic must carry out its discussions in a manner free from coercion (Parkinson, 2003). Those conducting deliberative processes seek to make them independent through providing information which is as 'neutral' as possible, through using moderators and organisers removed from the question at hand. In a citizens' jury the construction of a charge or a question is particularly open to manipulation by those in positions of power, leading to the strong recommendation that jury agendas should be constructed by a steering group consisting of relevant stakeholders and outside bodies (Coote & Lenaghan, 1997; Wakeford, 2002). There is evidence that citizens' juries have been manipulated or their decisions avoided and ignored by decision makers (Delap, 2001) and this is far less likely to happen if a wide number of decision makers take ownership of the construction of the charge and agenda (Clarke et al, 2000).

Policy effectiveness

The evidence about the affects of citizens' juries on policy decisions are mixed. McIver found in her analysis of some early juries that citizen jury recommendations had prioritised and added weight to particular issues rather than suggesting radical alternatives (1997). Policy makers interviewed as part of evaluations have found their conclusions useful and constructive (Barnes, 1999). An evaluation of jury processes in Scotland demonstrated that if the right local stakeholders were on board and if a question was seen to be relevant then jury recommendations would be acted upon. However, if an issue was not directly important to them, local decision makers were very good at avoiding taking action (Delap, 2001; Clarke et al, 2000).

It can be said that the process is constructed to encourage policy makers to answer to a group of citizens in a public manner. This in itself represents a step towards dialogue between local people and local agencies which a more deliberative approach demands. However, when agencies are not grounded in participation and dialogue, and when there is not enough local pressure, it is easy enough for them to ignore the conclusions of citizens.

Community ownership

While jurors and those immediately involved in the process have felt some sense of trust in the process it is difficult to assess the extent to which this is replicated in the wider community. Unlike conventional research, citizens' juries are public events – the process and the findings are publicised and a certain amount of observation is invited. Many juries have received a great deal of publicity.[8] However, the breadth, depth and length of this public awareness is difficult to analyse and very little evidence exists about whether increased trust between communities and local bodies continues once a jury has finished. Some commentators have suggested that the one-off nature of a jury together with the sense that it is owned by a particular agency such as a health authority decreases its legitimacy in the eyes of local people (Mort and Kashefi, 2002).

Increasing legitimacy: some recommendations

I have suggested that a deliberative process gains its legitimacy through the respect it can gain from local decision makers and the trust it can create in local communities. The citizens' jury has gone some way towards this but there are several ways the process can be made more robust and trustworthy:

Citizens juries as part of a process

It is important to see citizens' juries as one part in a process of involvement and discussion which is particularly suited to some questions and to some points on the decision making scale (Cabinet Office, 2001). It is true that for some public bodies the use of a jury have appeared to herald a new way of thinking about their consultation and relationship with the public. Consultation needs to be embedded into the culture of an organisation before it can be guaranteed that a citizens' jury can be used appropriately.

Creating a more public event

Allowing observers to watch some of the process has often enhanced the open nature of the citizens' jury. For practical reasons this can only be a small number of people. Experiments with running parallel internet juries and with filming juries directly onto an internet site so that they can be watched in progress have proved encouraging.[9] The use of electronic media represents a powerful possibility for creating a truly public process.[10]

Creating wider ownership

The steering group is the very minimum required to ensure independence. More importantly is a sense of ownership from local agencies and from local communities. In its original form the citizens' jury was 'commissioned' by a body such as a health authority which then answered its recommendations. There were two problems with this which practitioners have been attempting to rectify. Firstly that, if a jury is given a degree of freedom, their recommendations are relevant to more than one agency. In a pilot process in Scotland, 'stakeholder juries' worked in tandem with citizens juries to create action around different recommendations (Clarke et al, 2001). To a certain extent this was successful (Delap, 2001). But the more serious charge against juries is that they are owned by those in power, not by communities and those on the juries. This has led to practitioners experimenting in multi-agency juries on controversial topics (Wakeford, 2002), and looking at how to 'ground' citizens' juries in local communities, led principally by local community groups (Mort and Kashefi, 2002).

Conclusions: extending deliberative participation in the NHS

As the NHS moves into an era of increased local control there is a great need for robust participative approaches. The citizens jury experiment and the deliberative process has lessons for health related decision making bodies which need to gain local legitimacy and involve local people in a meaningful way. Those wishing to extend participation clearly face a number of barriers. For example:

A participative culture

Time and again studies conclude that bodies which make decisions about health must be more strategic in their approach to participation (National Consumer Council, 2002). The application of citizens' juries demonstrates that robust open processes need to be created within organisations to enable them to have the capacity and the willingness to involve local people.

Extending knowledge about appropriateness

In addition, when asked about the barriers to using more deliberative methods lack of knowledge about the possibilities is still a problem in many bodies.[11] It appears many policy makers go with well-known and established methods because of a lack of understanding about the range of methods and their suitability for different circumstances.

Working towards local ownership

Finally, too often structures are set up which are seen as either owned by policy makers *or* by communities. Creating bodies, which are both relevant to local policy makers and important to local communities, is a major challenge for those interested in extending participation.

The citizens' jury represents a brave attempt to instil some of the principles of deliberation into decision-making bodies in the UK. They have proved that it is possible to have robust, trustworthy mechanisms which include citizens in the complex health policy making. In order to make these more than a series of one-off experiments the principles of fair reasonable open dialogue need to be enshrined across the entire health service.

Notes

1. There has not been a complete record of all UK juries. This figure relies on the author's knowledge of a range of juries.
2. This case involved a child with leukaemia who's father disagreed with consultants about the necessity of treating her condition with a second bone marrow transplant. It illustrated the difficulties of prioritising healthcare particularly when the media became involved. See Ham & Pickard, 1998.
3. It would be true to say that the interest in promoting more local involvement had begun with the Local Voices recommendations of the early 1990s. See NHS Management Board, 1992.
4. New mechanisms are being put into place such as Patients Panels which are diverting attention from one-off consultations. See www.DoH.gov.uk.
5. Some practitioners prefer evening sittings to make the jury as convenient as possible for working people – see DIY jury project at www.peals.ncl.ac.uk
6. For instance user groups such as the Skye and Lochalsh young carers group or the Lambeth young people's parliament use many

deliberative approaches in their work. See Institute for Public Policy Research (IPPR), 2003 for further examples.

7. A citizens jury costs roughly between £20–40,000 plus time input from officers at the commissioning body. This includes recruitment costs, paying for moderators and outside organisers, setting up steering groups and collecting and collating information, and paying juror expenses.

8. For instance, a citizens' jury held in Belfast in 1999 commissioned by the Eastern Health and Social Services Board and Council received a great deal of attention from local medial – see Barnes, 1999 and Parkinson, 2002.

9. In a recent jury on genetically modified food the jury could be observed through an internet site as it was in progress. Viewers were encouraged to comment on the proceedings and at one point an interjection by email actually corrected some of the discussion in process. See www.food.gov.uk for the full jury proceedings. However, the extent to which such outside comments can be fed into the process has not been addressed.

10. In the USA several large deliberative events have been enhanced by the use of electronic methods. Their use in a small jury forum is more questionable. See www.americaspeaks.com.

11. This observation comes from interviews carried out by the author for Opinion Leader Research for a paper to be published later in 2003. See www.opinionleader.co.uk for further details.

References

Barnes, M. (1999) *Building a Deliberative Democracy, An evaluation of two citizens' juries*, IPPR, London.

Bryan, S., Roberts, T., Heginbotham, C. and McCallum, A. (1999) *Public Involvement in Health Care Priority Setting: an economic perspective*.

Cabinet Office (2002) *Viewfinder: a policy makers guide to public involvement*, available from the Cabinet Office website.

Clarke et al (2000) *Using People's Juries in Social Inclusion Partnerships: Guidance for SIPs*, Scottish Executive, Area Regeneration Division.

Clarke et al (2001) *People's Juries, Stakeholder Juries and Inter-Jury Fora in Social Inclusion Partnerships: a pilot project*, Scottish Executive Central Research Unit.

Combe, V., Delap, C. and Lenaghan, J. (1999) 'Rationing and Public Involvement: what have we learned?' unpublished discussion paper, IPPR, London.

Cooper, L., Coote, A., Davies, A. and Jackson, C. (1995) *Voices off: Tackling the democratic deficit in health*, IPPR, London,

Coote, A. and Lenaghan, J. (1997) Citizens' Juries: Theory into practice, IPPR, London.

Crosby, N. (1995) 'Citizens Juries, One solution for difficult environmental questions', in Renn, O., Webler, T. and Wiedermann, P. (eds) *Fairness and competence in citizen participation*, Dordecht: Kluwer.

Delap, C. 'Citizens' Juries, an overview of the UK experience' in PLA Notes 2001, Special Edition, 40, IIED (www.iied.org).

Dienel, P. and Renn, O. (1995) 'Planning cells: a gate to "fractal" mediation' in Renn, O., Webler, T. and Wiedermann, P. (eds) *Fairness and competence in citizen participation*, Dordecht: Kluwer.

Dunkerley, D. and Glasner, P. (1998) 'Empowering the Public: Citizens juries and the new genetic technologies', *Critical Public Health*, 8, 181–192.

Fishkin, J. (1995) *The Voice of the People, Public Opinion and Democracy*, New Haven: Yale University Press.

Fishkin, J, (1997) Appendix to *The Voice of the People, Public Opinion and Democracy* 2nd Edition, New Haven: Yale University Press.

Font, J. (ed.) (2001) *Ciudadanos y decisiones públicas*, University of Barcelona.

Ham, C. and Pickard, S. (1998) 'The Tragic Case of Child B', The Kings Fund, London.

Harrison, S. and Mort, M. (1999) 'Healthcare users, the public and the consultation industry', in Ling, T. (ed.) *Reforming Healthcare by Consent: Involving those who matter*, Oxford: Radcliffe Medical Press.

IDEA (2002) online evaluation framework: www.idea.gov.uk/bestvalue

IPPR (2003) *The IPPR/Guardian Public Involvement Awards 2003*, see www.ippr.org.uk.

Lenaghan, J. (1999) 'Involving the public in rationing decisions. The experience of citizens juries', *Health Policy*, 49(1–2): 45–61.

Lowndes, V. and Stoker, G. et al (1998) *Guidance on Enhancing public participation in local government: a research report to the Department of Environment, Transport and the Regions*, DETR, London.

Marsh, R., Rowe, G. and Frewer, L. (2001) *Public Participation Methods: Evolving and Operationalising an evaluation framework. Developing and testing a toolkit for evaluating the success of public participation exercises.* Report to the Department of Health, Institute of Food Research, Norwich see www.doh.gov.uk/risk.htm.

Mort, M. and Kashefi, E. (2001) 'Grounded Citizens' Juries: a tool for health improvement?' Paper given to Regione Emilia-Romagna Conference on Health Improvement Plans: institutions and citizens listen to each other, Bologna 2001.

McIver, S. (1997) *An Evaluation of the King's Fund Citizens' Juries Programme*, University of Birmingham, Health Services Management Centre.

McIver, S. (1998) *Healthy Debate: an independent evaluation of citizens' juries in health settings*, King's Fund, London.

National Consumer Council (2002) 'Involving consumers in healthcare case study for the Involving Consumers Project', see www.ncc.org.uk.

New, B. (1999) *A Good Enough Service Values Trade-offs and the NHS*, IPPR, London.

NHS Management Services (1992) Local Voices, the views of local people in purchasing for health, London.

Parkinson, J. (2003) 'Why deliberation? The use of deliberation by new public managers', Paper given to Political Studies Association Conference, University of Leicester, 15–17 April 2003.

Public Administration Select Committee (2001) *Public Participation: issues and innovations, Vol. 1: report and proceedings of the committee*, House of commons, London.

Renn, O. and Webler, T. (1995) 'A brief primer on Participation: philosophy and practice', in Renn, O., Webler, T. and Wiedermann, P. (eds) *Fairness and competence in citizen participation*, Dordecht: Kluwer.

Rogers, B. (2003) 'Reality Spoils a good story about reforms', *Financial Times*, June 17th.

Smith, G. and Wales, C. (2000) 'Citizens' juries and deliberative democracy', *Political Studies*, 48(1): 51–65.

Stewart, J. (1996) *Further Innovations in Democratic Practice*, Institute of Local Government Studies, University of Birmingham.

Stewart, J., Kendall, L. and Coote, A. (1994) *Citizens' Juries*, IPPR, London.

Wakeford, T. (2002) 'Citizens Juries a radical alternative for social research', Social research update 37 Summer, Dept Sociology, University of Surrey.

Women's Unit (1998) Jury Conclusion and recommendations (unpublished report).

7

'On the shoulders of Giants': Putting the Quality into Qualitative Methods in 'Consumer' Research

Jennifer Burr

Introduction

This chapter provides a brief overview of the literature on quality assurance in qualitative research, in particular the notion of 'checklists' for quality in qualitative research. The backdrop to this chapter is the use of qualitative methods used to access the views of users[1] of health and social care. Debate about whether criteria should be applied to assessing the quality of qualitative research, and if so, what criteria should comprise of, is controversial.[2] Controversy also includes debate about what qualitative research is and the variety of different approaches included within qualitative research. The standpoint taken here however, is that it is possible to recognise poor qualitative research which fails to present enough information about the methods and analysis. This is not to argue that the application of a checklist to research would necessarily produce 'good' qualitative research. As Barbour argues reducing qualitative research to a list of technical procedures, however extensive, is overly prescriptive and results in 'the tail wagging the dog' (2001).

Therefore, this chapter will not be producing another checklist for qualitative research.[3] Rather, the aim is to discuss and illustrate the importance to qualitative research of *epistemology* through an analysis of methodological critiques. As the sociologist Robert Merton argued, we should stand *On the Shoulders of Giants* (1965) who have gone before us if we are to learn and not repeat the mistakes of our predecessors. The discussion in this chapter will draw upon the work of Murphy et al. *Qualitative Research Methods in Health Technology Assessment: a review of the literature*. In addition, the chapter also draws upon the author's work as part of the CHePAS Scoping study[4] which featured recommendations for future research methodologies used to elicit users' views of health care, including a large section on recommendations for qualitative research. The recommendations were based upon a specific but detailed audit of relevant qualitative research in peer-reviewed journals. The team concluded that, with reference to qualitative research 'There is a need for more understanding of the research process and the need for analytical rigour in conducting and reporting qualitative research' (2001, p. 72).

What is qualitative research

Qualitative research has different objectives, asks different questions and provides different answers to those of other types of research (see also Chapter 11). Qualitative methods are not concerned with issues of how many people in a given area experience a type of illness or use a type of service provision. Rather the use of qualitative research can help in understanding what it feels like to suffer from an illness or what individuals think about a particular service.

Sykes et al (1992) summarise the use of qualitative research methodologies as providing 'direct access' to the experiences and perceptions of health care users. Qualitative research has the potential to provide a more in-depth understanding of the behaviour of individuals.

Qualitative research also has the potential to help people feel 'actively involved' in the provision of health care services rather than the passive providers of information. Qualitative research has the capacity to make people feel more important and that their views are valued.

Qualitative research can give a 'voice' to people who are traditionally marginalised, including ethnic minorities and people with disabilities (see Chapter 10).

Qualitative research is particularly useful in providing information on sensitive issues including the intimate aspects of being cared for and which individuals may find difficult to outline in other research methods.

Qualitative research methods have strengths and weaknesses and are not suitable for all types of research. They are time consuming especially in comparison to more quantitative methods. The limitations of qualitative methods are that they are not generalisable to a wider community in the way that large scale surveys may be seen to be. Qualitative research involves interpretation and acknowledges a subjective element in the research process. The implications are that qualitative researchers have frequently been asked to account for their work in terms of scientific value (see further discussion of this point, and the importance to qualitative research of subjectivity, in Chapter 11).

Qualitative research is characterised by epistemological diversity and the review of existing qualitative research accessing users views, which was conducted, by CHePAS, for the NHS Service Delivery and Organisation (SDO), revealed that most fell broadly into what Reicher (2000) has termed as *experimental*. Essentially it is qualitative research that aims to gain a better understanding of user's experiences and ways of thinking about their care. This is in contrast to *discursive* qualitative research that is concerned with the role of language or power in the construction of reality. Experimental research assumes that language is a reflection of understanding and can therefore be used to mirror what people think. The literature review also revealed that the most common qualitative methods used in eliciting users views were interviews, including semi-structured and in-depth, individual interviews and group or focus group interviews.

Given the predominance of the use of individual interviews and focus groups in accessing users' views a brief definition is provided below:

Individual interviews

Interviews can be structured to varying degrees of formality and tend to be described as semi-structured. The notion of an 'unstructured' interview is misleading as no interview is devoid of some form of structure (Britten, 1995). Semi-structured interviews consist of a loose structure of open-ended questions that guide the respondent through the area under exploration. The interviewee may diverge from the loose structure in order to pursue some aspect of the respondent's comment in more detail. However, and as discussed below, the terminology used to describe the format of individual interviews is not always clear. The interviewer requires considerable skill in order to successfully explore the interviewee's frame of reference and not impose their own assumptions. The implications for accessing users' views and the role of the interviewer are discussed in more detail below (also see Chapter 11).

The focus group has also gained in popularity in accessing users' views.

The focus group

One simple definition of a focus group is that it involves 8 to 12 individuals who discuss a particular topic under the direction of a moderator who promotes interaction and assures that the discussion remains on the topic (Stewart and Shamdasani, 1990, p. 10).

The focus group can work in conjunction with other methods, or it can stand alone as a self-contained method in its own right (Morgan, 1988). The goal in using focus groups is essentially that of learning about participants' experiences and perspectives (Morgan, 1988).

The use of focus groups provides rich and diverse data, validated distinctively through social rather than personal processes (Albrecht et al, 1993). It is the collective identity provided in the focus group, which is likely to result in data reflecting the experiences of the community as a whole, which makes focus groups an ideal research method for exploring the views that different groups of health or social care user may have.

The collective nature of the focus group allows responses to be placed in their proper context rather than forcing responses into an individualistic and isolated framework which the researcher may consider appropriate (Merton, 1956). In this sense the focus group is more likely to encourage 'emic' categories of knowledge, that is knowledge grounded in everyday life through locally relevant terms (Stewart and Shamdasani, 1990).

However, as discussed below, the use of the focus group as been somewhat distorted in accessing users' views and there is a large degree of misunderstanding about the scope of focus groups.

The range and use of criteria for assessing qualitative research

Even the most cursory glance at any peer reviewed journal reveals the popularity of qualitative methods for accessing the views of users of health and social care services. It is possible that the popularity of qualitative methods is that they purport to reflect the 'voice' of the health and social care user and therefore, are increasingly recognised as methods for gaining insight into user's experiences and perceptions of their health care.

However, it is also evident that the use of qualitative methods and reporting of qualitative findings is, in many instances, poorly understood and of a poor quality (CHePAS, 2001). Whilst there is a comprehensive range of texts which provide clear guidance on conducting and analysing qualitative methods (for example Bryman & Burgess, 1994) there is an evident lack of analytical rigour in the application of these methods in health and social care research and in some nursing research in particular.

It has been argued that the search for criteria for assessing good qualitative research stands in direct opposition to what qualitative research stands for. For example, Smith (1984) argues that qualitative research represents a distinct paradigm from quantitative which is predicated upon what can be defined as an anti-realist standpoint. This involves an understanding of the philosophical position which argues that reality is dependent upon the mind of the observer. Therefore, such a position runs contrary to the idea of an objective standpoint which might be used as a criterion against which research findings might be judged. This position however, raises serious doubts, for some, about the contribution to health and social care practice made by qualitative research (Murphy et al, 1998).

Among the qualitative researchers who accept the importance of identifying a criteria for assessing qualitative research there are substantial variability in the criteria proposed. A summary of these positions is provided by Murphy et al. In their comprehensive HTA review the authors go on to reject the anti-realist argument of the likes of Smith and argue for a middle of the road approach advocated by Hammersly (1990). Hammersly (1990) argues that the function of research is to produce knowledge which has relevance to public concern and that therefore, there are two criteria against which such research can be assessed: validity and relevance. Following Hammersly Murphy et al propose that the most appropriate criteria for evaluating qualitative research are validity and relevance and that, for research to inform development 'we must, first and foremost, have some confidence that their findings are true. Likewise their relevance to the concerns identified by [HTA] commissioners must be clear' (178, 1998). However, Hammersley cautions against defining relevance in terms which are too narrow. Silverman (1993), for example, has argued that it is not always in researcher's interests to accept uncritically a research problem identified by practitioners. In other words, it cannot always be assumed that the problem identified by practitioners is the problem which needs to be addressed. For example, Health Policy relating to young pregnancy has been 'problem' targeted focussing upon the dominant health discourse, and a negative view of (young) female sexuality and diverting attention away from the wider contexts (Ingham & Kirkland, 1997). There is evidence that few young people contextualise their early sexual experiences within a medical discourse. Therefore, there is a need to reframe problem identification within the social contexts in which risk-taking behaviour occurs.

Validity and reliability

There remains confusion over the value of the terms validity and reliability when applied to qualitative research although these concepts appeared frequently in the studies reviewed for the CHePAS study. Respondent validation has been suggested as a means of establishing the validity of findings of qualitative research by a number of authors (see for example Guba and Lincoln, 1989). The approach most commonly adopted is that the validation of the researcher's analysis is judged by those studied and agreed as adequately representing their views. Given the current focus on consumerism, respondent validation has political appeal. However, respondent validation cannot be treated as an unproblematic test of validity (Bloor, 1983). As qualitative researchers continue to argue, responses from respondents are situational. Member checks may offer additional evidence which are still open to interpretation. As Mays and Pope point out, researchers seek to provide an overview whereas respondents have individual concerns, and this can result in apparently discrepant accounts (2000).

Respondent validation can be particularly valuable in action research projects, where researchers work with participants on an ongoing basis to facilitate change (see Allan, 2001 in Chapter 10). However, the health services research reviewed by CHePAS, which purported to use respondent validation, involved a one-off data collection exercise, in which respondent validation may be more trouble than it is worth.

Validity and reliability through investigator validation, or triangulation, is a similar approach to respondent validation. For example, in a study which attempted to explore the complexities of the outpatient experience for recipients of care Somerset et al argued that : 'In order to enhance validity of the process of analysis, the researchers discussed their readings and codings and exchanged transcripts' (Somerset et al, 1999, p. 215).

There can be little doubt that the use triangulation may extend the comprehensiveness of a research study. However, triangulation as a form of validation is also open criticism. First, Silverman (1985, 1993) argues that the basis of triangulation is fundamentally misplaced in qualitative research as it attempts to overcome the context boundedness of data. Analysis in 'context' is in fact at the core of qualitative research and analysis. Second, attempts to gain validity through triangulation may result in researchers focusing their analyses on the the search for a single reality or truth. Silverman (1993) argues that multiple methods help to adjudicate between accounts, providing the researcher does not end up judging between these accounts.

Having established that member checks and triangulation are misplaced in qualitative research Murphy et al offer five principles on which judgements about the validity of qualitative research findings may be made. These five principles are described below and further substantiated by the CHePAS findings which are used to provide discrete examples taken from 'consumer' based qualitative research.

1. Clear exposition of data collection method

A basic premise of qualitative research is the recognition that data must be understood in relation to the context of their production. It is therefore, important that qualitative researchers create a record of the research process which should include, amongst other things, a clear exposition of the process of data collection, including 'details of the researcher's role within the research setting, the selection of informants within the setting, and the social conditions within which data were collected' (Murphy et al, 186).

Under this heading can also be added the need to provide a clear and comprehensive outline of the methods used. The CHePAS study revealed that, perhaps not surprisingly and as discussed above, that interviews were a popular method for eliciting user views and authors referred to different types of interview format. Semi-structured interviews were the mainstay of the interview format referred to in most studies, although terminology was also vague ('unstructured interviews', 'detailed interview' and 'open interview format' were referred to).

Focus groups were also popular and the mechanics and strengths and weaknesses of focus groups are well-documented, as outlined above. For example, in a study which explored the perceptions of psychiatric service users about their needs an appropriate use of focus groups was described to: 'promote a sense of collective remembering between group participants' (Jackson, 2000). In addition, Jackson described how a component of this collective nature would be that focus group members could 'challenge each other's views, so adding to the range of the data collected' (p. 379).

However, the concept of the focus group was also misapplied. For example, Dolan describes how focus groups were used 'to facilitate discussion between respondents' (p. 318, 1999). However, within this study the focus groups were highly structured with respondents being asked to rank hypothetical patient cases in terms of priorities and make separate sets of comparisons between patients. Distinct and comparable data would appear to be the required outcome of focus groups in this study rather than rich and diverse data. Dolan's use of the focus group is questionable. The processes are more akin to the Nominal Group Technique (NGT) in that the authors are reporting agreement in group discussion and are attempting to reach a consensus of views rather than explore diversity.

2.   Clear exposition of process of data analysis

Increasingly, authors have rightly criticised qualitative researchers for their failure to provide a clear outline of how their findings have been derived from the data collected. Melia (1997) has derided explanations of analysis as tinged with 'near mysticism'. An outline should be provided and include the process by which data have been coded and categorised and the way in which conclusions have been drawn from the data collected.

a) Coding and categorising data

The use of 'Grounded Theory' techniques emerged commonly as descriptions of both method and analysis in the studies on users' views reviewed by the CHePAS team. It is acknowledged that the original Grounded Theory technique as outlined by Glaser and Strauss (1967) is particularly complex. It can be a matter of judgement as to how far authors who make claims to be conducting 'grounded theory' actually are. However, it was clear that few, if any of the studies reviewed by the CHePAS team were utilising grounded theory but rather using a process of identifying and generating themes and subthemes which were coded.

Bryman and Burgess have criticised the use of grounded theory as 'an approving bumper sticker' invoked to confer academic respectability rather than as a helpful description of the strategy used in analysis (1994). Similarly, Melia (997) claims that most researchers use a pragmatic variant, whereby they identify new themes from the data alongside those that could have been anticipated from the outset. In the absence of an attempt to systematically analyse the commonalities and contradictions reflected in the data, many researchers produce an artificially neat and tidy account that is descriptive rather than analytical. The reader is expected to take it on trust that theory somehow emerges from the data without being offered an explanation of how theoretical insights have been established.

b) Drawing conclusions from the data

The CHePAS study argued for the importance of providing examples of data to illustrate analytical procedures. The use of quotations provides the opportunity for the reader to appraise the fit between the data and the authors understanding and use of that data (Elliot, 1999).

For example, Paterson and Britten (2000) provided a clear example of the reporting of qualitative data. In a study using semi-structured interviews the authors explored the views of people with asthma about the organisation of asthma care in general practice. They quote the mother of a six-year old girl with asthma who is commenting on 'expert knowledge and therapeutic relationships':

> 'If she was fine I don't have a problem with seeing the asthma nurse. I mean, I don't if she was fine, but if she was really poorly, then I would rather prefer to see the doctor...I mean, I know the asthma nurse could do that as well, but, I don't know, there's something about a doctor [laugh], there's something about a doctor that gives you the confidence to, you know deal with the situation' (p. 302, 2000).

The use of qualitative data are required to provide evidence of the process of analysis. A particularly poor example of the use of data as evidence is provided in the work of McGonagle and Gentle (1996). In this study the authors are attempting to discover the reasons for non-attendance at a mental health day hospital. In elaborating upon how their respondents had described a lack of an individual approach to their care the authors state that 'The general feeling was that they [clients] were offered a set pro-gramme regardless of their expressed problems' (p. 63) The authors then quote respondents or a respondent thus:

> 'It was as though I was a number, a nobody, and one was just put here and there
>
> They treat us all as one
>
> They suggested social groups, but I know they don't help' (p. 63, 1996).

It is not clear whether these are multiple responses or from the same person. In addition there is no indication of the age or gender of the respondent. Such information is important in grounding the findings of qualitative research. It is ironic that the respondent is complaining about being 'a nobody' and is still a 'nobody' in the treatment by the researcher. Moreover, these responses could have been predicted from the onset.

3.   Reflexivity

Within the quantitative tradition the emphasis is upon eliminat-ing the impact of the researcher upon the research findings. However, researchers within the qualitative tradition acknowledge that the research process and analysis are invariably shaped by the social world within which they are produced (see Chapter 11). Essentially, reflexivity means a sensitivity to how the researcher's presence within the research setting has contributed to the data collected and the impact of their a priori assumptions upon the analysis. In other words, the credibility of research findings is enhanced when the researcher makes explicit the personal and theoretical standpoints which they bring to the research process. For example, with reference to the CHePAS findings, researchers maintained a concern with validity without the consideration of reflexivity. The exception was Powell et al (1994) who stated that the process of analysis entailed 'self reflexivity' (p. 200). Unfortunately, however, there is no discussion as to how this was achieved so the statement was somewhat meaningless.

The concern over the lack of methodological rigor has been echoed elsewhere. In a review of 29 papers, which reported to use qualitative methods in researching issues in general practice, Hoddinott and Pill (1997) concluded that these papers often lacked explicit methodological detail about the relationship between the interviewer and the respondent.

4. Attention to negative cases

Attention to negative cases can loosely be defined as the conscientious search for and presentation of data that are inconsistent with the emerging analysis. The careful study of negative cases allows the researcher the opportunity to challenge and refine their analyses. Closely related to attention to negative cases is the tendency for the qualitative researcher to limit themselves to single studies which limit the search for negative evidence. Murphy et al therefore, argue that 'one of the criteria by which qualitative research should be judged is the extent to which the researchers have built upon previous knowledge in their work and their success in connecting their findings with previous knowledge' (p. 192).

Within this context there is clearly a requirement to recognise the differences between rigorous and well-designed qualitative research and attempts to supplement quantification with more open-ended interviews. For example: McGonagle (1996) report that 'Forty-two per cent (n = 6) experienced attending the day hospital as traumatic because they felt they were not listened to' (p. 63). Clearly there has been no consideration of negative cases and the data are presented as from a crude survey. Qualitative methods are not about homogenising responses but about muddle and complexity.

5. Fair dealing

The commitment to multiple perspectives, upon which the qualitative tradition is predicated, has a range of implications for assessing the validity of qualitative research findings. In particular, multiple perspectives suggests that the researcher must attempt to do justice to the range of perspectives and not present the perspective of one group as the objective truth about the phenomenon in question. The issue of partisanship in qualitative research has elicited a somewhat polarised response. On the one hand there are authors who have argued that research is always morally and politically partisan (Becker, 1967). The 'underdog' perspective in qualitative research has a long history but more recently, a concern has emerged that the perspective of the underdog fails to represent the interactive character of social life. On the other hand, therefore, is the perspective that the powerful and the privileged also have something to say and to exclude these views is little more than, in the words of Dingwall, 'muck-raking journalism' (1992, p. 172). It is a key concern however, that even with an increasing political emphasis upon the role of the 'consumer' in health care, that there remains distinct groups whose voices remain unheard. This include: children, groups with some mental illnesses, the elderly and some ethnic minority groups, especially those for whom English is not their first language (see Chapter 10).

What is evident however, is that the emphasis upon 'consumers' in health care assumes a generalised conception of 'consumers' which is uncritically accepted within health policy (see Chapter 2 and Introduction). Atkinson has warned of the dangers of 'romanticising' respondents' accounts (1997). Certainly, there has been a tendency in 'consumer' research to treat the 'consumer' as unproblematic and as a single authoritative voice. From this perspective the 'consumer' is likely to have their own agendas and their 'voices' should not be treated as unpartisan. In this sense, the rise of the 'new' consumer within health care (see chapter 2) serves to further marginalise minority groups.

Conclusions

Murphy et al provide us with a useful framework from which to asses the quality of qualitative research. The CHePAS study also made the following recommendations for the use of qualitative research in accessing users views:

i)   Making explicit aims and objectives and research questions for exploration

ii) Providing a clear and comprehensive outline of the methods used
iii) Providing a clear outline of whom is conducting the research and the relationship between the interviewed and the interviewee.
iv) The process of analysis should be explicit.

Finally, the CHePAS study also cautions that the use of 'grounded theory' has become a short cut for a process of identifying themes and coding.

The risk of any form of 'checklist' for qualitative research is that they are interpreted as 'technical fixes' (Barbour, 2001). It has in fact been argued that a particular advantage of qualitative methods is that 'they do not require the degree of technical skill needed to produce and interpret statistical data' (May, 1995). There is the need to challenge the assumption that qualitative research can be conducted by anyone, regardless of their training, and that conducting and interpreting qualitative data does not require skill. What becomes evident from a consideration of the literature on the subject of checklists, and the review of the CHePAS study, is the overall need for a broad understanding of qualitative research design and data analysis including an emphasis upon the importance of reflexivity (see Chapter 11). Such an understanding is not to be captured with the use of a checklist. Without a theoretical basis, as Paul Atkinson has argued, using qualitative methods 'would be like my saying to Angus Clarke (a clinical geneticist), I'll just do a bit of DNA sequencing using some kitchen equipment' (1999, p. 11).

Without productive ideas and theoretical perspectives to drive them qualitative methods will not generate systematic knowledge about the social world that the researcher purports to reflect when using them. Without an understanding of the theoretical basis of qualitative research we run the risk of compromising the unique contribution that qualitative research can make to improving health and social services.

Notes

1. The term 'user' is a preference to 'consumer'. Please see introduction.

2.   See Chapter 11 in this volume.
3.   There are already a number of criteria in existence within the fields of sociology (for example the criteria for evaluation of qualitative research adopted by the Medical Sociology Group of the British Sociological Association) and psychology (Willig, 2001, chapter 9) (see also http://www.iphrp.salford.ac.uk/cochrane/biblio.htm for an overview).
4.   Consumer Health Psychology at ScHARR (2001) Eliciting users' views of the processes of health care: a scoping study: NHS R&D Service Delivery and Organisation. (See http://www.sdo.lshtm.ac.uk/research-methods.htm)

References

Albrecht, T., Johnson, G. and Walther, J. (1993) Understanding Communication Processes in Focus Groups. In Morgan, D. (ed.) *Successful Focus Groups: Advancing the State of the Art*, London: Sage.

Allan, K. (2001) *Communication and consultation: Exploring ways for staff to involve people with dementia in developing services*, The Policy Press.

Atkinson, P. (1997) Narrative turn or blind alley? *Qualitative Health Research*, 7: 325–344.

Atkinson, P. (1999) Changing perceptions on the politics and ethics of qualitative research. *Qualitative research: a vital resource for ethical health care* (Volume 2) Proceedings of the conference organised by the UK Forum for Health Care, Law and Ethics, London: Wellcome Trust.

Barbour, R. (2001) Checklists for improving rigour in qualitative research: a case of the tail wagging the dog? *British Medical Journal*, 322: 1115–1117.

Becker, H. (1967) Whose side are we on? *Social Problems*, 14: 239–48.

Bloor, M. (1983) Notes on member validation. In Emerson, R. (ed.) *Contemporary field research: A collection of Readings*, Boston: Little, Brown.

Britten, N. (1995) Qualitative Interviews in Medical Research, *British Medical Journal*, 311: 251–253.

Bryman, A. and Burgess, R. (1994) (eds) *Analysing Qualitative Data*, London: Routledge.

Burns, N. and Grove, S. (1993) *The Practice of Nursing Research: Conduct, Critique and Utilization*, Philadelphia: WB Saunders.

CHePAS (Consumer Health Psychology at ScHARR) (2001) *Eliciting Users' views of the processes of Health care: A Scoping Study*, The NHS Service Delivery and Organisation (SDO).

Denzin, N. (1970) *The Research Act*, Englewood Cliffs, NJ: Prentice Hall.

Dingwall, R. (1992) Don't mind him – he's from Barcelona: qualitative methods in health studies. In: Daly, J., McDonald, I. and Wilks, E. (eds) *Researching Health Care*, London: Tavistock/Routledge.

Dolan, P., Cookson, R. and Ferguson, B. (1999) Effect of discussion and deliberation on the public's views of priority setting in health care: a Focus group study, *British Medical Journal*, 318: 916–918.

Elliott, R., Fischer, C. and Rennie, D. (1999) Evolving Guidelines for publication of qualitative research studies in psychology and related fields, *British Journal of Clinical Psychology*, 38: 215–29.

Glaser, B. and Strauss, A. (1967) *The Discovery of Grounded Theory: Strategies for Qualitative Research*, New York: Aldine.

Guba, E. and Lincoln, Y. (1989) *Fourth Generation Evaluation*, Newbury Park, CA: Sage.

Hammersley, M. (1990) *Reading Ethnographic Research*, New York: Longman.

Hoddinott, P. and Pill, R. (1997) A review of recently published qualitative research in general practice. More methodological questions than answers? *Family Practice*, 14: 313–319.

Ingham, R. and Kirkland, D. (1997) Discourses and sexual health: providing for young people. In Yardley, L. (ed.) *Material Discourses of Health and Illness*, London: Routledge.

Jackson, S. and Stevenson, C. (2000) What do people need psychiatric and mental health nurses for? *Journal of Advanced Nursing*, 31: 378–388.

Janesick, V. (1994) The dance of qualitative research design: metaphor, methodolatory and meaning. In Denzin, N. and Lincoln, Y. (eds) *Handbook of qualitative Research*, Thousand Oaks, CA: Sage.

Kitzinger, J. (1994) 'The Methodology of Focus Groups: The Importance of Interaction Between Research Participants'. In *Sociology of Health and Illness*, 16: 103–121.

May, C. (1995) More semi than structured? Some problems with qualitative research methods, *Nurse Education Today*, 16: 189–192.

Mays, N. and Pope, C. (2000) Assessing quality in qualitative research, *British Medical Journal*, 320: 50–52.

McGonagle, I. and Gentle, J. (1996) Reasons for non-attendance at a day hospital for people with enduring mental illness: the clients' perspective, *Journal of Psychiatric and Mental Health Nursing*, 3: 61–66.

Melia, K.M. (1997) Producing 'plausible stories': interviewing student nurses. In: Miller, G., Dingwall, R. (eds) *Context and Method in Qualitative Research*, London: Sage, 26–36.

Merton, R., Fisk, M. and Kendall, P. (1956) *The Focused Interview: A Manual of Problems and Procedures*, Glencoe: The Free Press.

Merton, R. (1965) *On the Shoulders of Giants: A Shandean Postscript*, New York: Free Press.

Morgan, D. (1988) *Focus Groups as Qualitative Research*, London: Sage.

Murphy, E., Dingwall, R., Greatbatch, D., Parker, S. and Watson, P. (1998) *Qualitative research methods in health technology assessment: a review of the literature*, Health Techno Assessment: 2: (16).

Paterson, C. and Britten, N. (2000) Organising primary health care for people with asthma: the patient's perspective, *British Journal of General Practice*, 50: 299–303.

128 *Researching Health Care Consumers*

Powell, J., Lovelock, R., Bray, J. and Philp, I. (1994) Involving consumers in assessing service quality: benefits of using a qualitative approach, *Qual. Health Care*, 3: 199–202.

Reicher, S. (2000) Against methodollatry: Some comments on Elliott, Fischer, and Rennie. *British Journal of Clinical Psychology*, 39: 1–6.

Silverman, D. (1985) *Qualitative Methodology and Sociology*, Aldershot: Gower.

Silverman, D. (1993) *Interpreting Qualitative Data: Methods for Analysing Talk, Text and Interaction*, London: Sage.

Smith, J. (1984) The problem of criteria for judging interpretive inquiry, *Educational Evaluation and Policy Analysis*, 6: 379–91.

Somerset, M., Faulkner, A., Shaw, A., Dunn, L. and Sharp, D. (1999) Obstacles on the path to a primary-care led National health Service: Complexities of outpatient care, *Social Science and Medicine*, 48: 213–225.

Stewart, D. and Shamdasani, P. (1990) *Focus Groups: Theory and Practice*, London: Sage.

Sykes, W., Collins, M., Hunter, J., Popay, J. and Williams, G. (1992) *Listening to local Voices: A Guide to Research*, Nuffield Institute for Health Services Studies.

Willig, C. (2001) *Introducing Qualitative Research in Psychology: Adventures in Theory and Method*, Buckingham: Open University Press.

8

The Role of Information Technology in Accessing Consumer Perspectives

Catherine Beverley and Andrew Booth

Introduction

Information Technology (IT) clearly offers diverse and expanded research opportunities (Sharf, 1999) in accessing consumer perspectives (Murray, 1995; Houston & Fiore, 1998; Gillespie, 1999). The terms 'user' and 'consumer' are used interchangeably throughout this chapter to denote individuals or groups of people who are, or have been, in contact with health services. This definition is based on Boote et al (2002) and Consumers in NHS Research (2000). Unlike many of the other terms available (e.g. client, lay person, etc.), both 'user' and 'consumer' are relatively neutral words that imply a two-way relationship between the researcher and participant. IT encompasses a wide range of technologies, but this chapter focuses on Internet-enabled applications, such as those facilitated by the World Wide Web (WWW) and electronic mail (email). IT has evolved from supporting the analysis of data (Posavac et al, 1981), to communicating research ideas and findings (Ehrenberger & Murray, 1998; Eysenbach &

Wyatt, 2002), and providing new approaches to conducting both quantitative and qualitative research (Lakeman, 1997). Information posted by consumers on the Internet may help to identify health beliefs, common topics, motives, information, and emotional needs of patients and point to areas where research is needed (Eysenbach & Wyatt, 2002).

This chapter provides an overview of published literature and outlines potential developments. It begins by analysing how technology already substitutes for traditional research methods, such as questionnaires, interviews and focus groups. Such a simple 'substitution' allows methods familiar to many researchers and users to be made more widely available. However, critics argue that these approaches seek merely to replicate (sometimes less favourably) established methods, and, in doing so, fail to capitalise on the real strengths of IT. Newer approaches (e.g. bulletin boards, electronic discussion groups, and Internet chat rooms) are then examined. The effect of technology on the researcher-consumer relationship is considered. The chapter concludes by suggesting possible future methodological contributions of IT to consumer health research.

Substituting IT for traditional methods of accessing consumer perspectives

Most proposed applications of IT seek to reproduce established research methodologies in a way that is facilitated, but not necessarily extended, by the technology. So, for example:

The questionnaire is translated into the electronic questionnaire, administered via a variety of routes, such as email (Kaufman, 1997; Schmidt, 1997; Mavis, 1998; Eley, 1999; Cooper, 2000; Lakeman, 2000).

The interview is conducted either asynchronously (separated in time, or 'offline') via email (Thach, 1995; Selwyn & Robson, 1998; Cooper, 2000), or synchronously (in real-time, or 'live') via audio or video links.

The focus group is enabled asynchronously via a mailing list discussion group or newsgroup, or synchronously using a chat room or virtual meeting room (Lakeman, 1997; Velikova et al, 1999; Schneider et al, 2002).

A Delphi process is achieved through successive rounds of staged email messages (Cabaniss, 2001).

The major IT methods

Electronic questionnaires

According to Murray (1995), the questionnaire is the most common method used on the Internet for data collection. It may be administered via a standalone computer (Kiesler & Sproull, 1986; Murrelle et al, 1992; Coomber, 1997; Gillespie, 1999; Heerwegh & Loosveldt, 2002), a touch screen interface (Lau et al, 1996; Velikova et al, 1999; Lofland et al, 2000), an email message or attachment (Chappel et al, 1999; Eley, 1999; Treadwell et al, 1999; Cooper, 2000; Lipsitz et al, 2001), or via a Web site or online discussion group (Bell & Kahn, 1996; Houston & Fiore, 1998; Davis, 1999; Cook et al, 2000; Conboy et al, 2001).

An online survey is inherently no more complex to develop than its traditional counterpart. The same basic process is followed: write the survey, direct it to the desired population, and interpret the data (Houston & Fiore, 1998). Many principles associated with good survey design for postal questionnaires similarly apply; a questionnaire should be relevant to the participant, short, and simple to follow (Murray, 1995; Edwards et al, 2002). (Some of the principles of good survey design are also outlined by Steven Bruster in Chapter 4 of this volume). However, additional factors that need to be considered when designing electronic surveys include; the need to bear in mind varying levels of IT expertise amongst the participants, and to avoid the use of tick boxes which can be problematic for the inexperienced computer user (Murray, 1995).

The use of electronic questionnaires is frequently reported in the literature, with many examples from the health field (Murray, 1995; Kim et al, 1997; Eley, 1999; Gillespie, 1999). Fischbacher et al (2000) identify 43 examples of the use of the Internet for health surveys. However, most of these cover the use of IT, the patients' experiences of particular conditions, research methods and health professionals' perceptions of the use of health services, rather than Internet-enabled surveys specifically designed to elicit the views of general users of health services or canvassing the opinions of those within a defined geographical location or community.

Example 1: The computerised questionnaire

Ryan et al (2002) tested the effect of the electronic mode of administration on the measurement properties of the Short Form-36 (SF-36) General Health Questionnaire. In a randomised cross-over design study, 79 healthy individuals and 35 chronic pain patients completed both electronic and paper versions of the SF-36. Participants completed the electronic version on a stand-alone computer. 77 per cent preferred the electronic SF-36, 7 per cent stated no preference and 22 per cent preferred the paper version. Completion time for the electronic SF-36 was slightly less, and there were no missing or problematical responses, whereas 44 per cent of participants had at least one missing or problem-atic response in the paper version. The authors concluded that the electronic SF-36 was equivalent in performance and more effective than the paper version.

Example 2: The email questionnaire

Through email, Lipsitz et al (2001) surveyed members of an Internet support group for emetophobia (fear of vomiting). Based on responses to a series of open-ended questions, a survey of 29 items was composed. This questionnaire was distributed by email to the 100 plus active mailgroup members by the List Server Co-ordinator. Fifty six completed surveys were returned to the co-ordinator who removed the email addresses and any other identifying information before forwarding the responses to the researchers.

Example 3: The WWW questionnaire

Conboy et al (2001) questioned middle-aged women (aged 35–49) regarding their current attitudes, beliefs, symptoms and treatment choices surrounding the climateric (menopause). 448 self-selecting visitors to the Women's Health Interactive Web site completed the 189-item Web-based survey. Findings were similar to those obtained using large randomised telephone survey methods. The authors concluded that the Internet was a reliable and convenient venue for gathering data regarding health issues.

Electronic interviews

There are several ways to conduct structured electronic interviews with perhaps the simplest and most effective being via email. Whereas email in electronic surveys directly replaces conventional mail, electronic interviewing makes use of the more interactive and immediate nature of email (Selwyn & Robson, 1998). Selwyn & Robson (1998) highlight generic advantages and disadvantages associated with electronic interviews (refer to Figure 8.1).

Example 4: The structured email interview

Surprisingly there are only a handful of examples of electronic interviews being used in practice (e.g. Foster, 1994; Murray, 1995). Murray (1995) conducted a number of interviews by email with subscribers to the Nursenet list. After inviting list-members to contact him, he conducted detailed interviews with five people from North America and Europe. A common set of questions was used to structure the initial stages with the interviews subsequently becoming unstructured.

Electronic discussion groups

Focus groups may be a time-effective method of eliciting the views of a large number of people. Unfortunately, face-to-face focus groups are often time-consuming to organise and costly to run (refer to Chapter 7). Electronic discussion groups may overcome these problems. Tse (1999) highlights advantages and disadvantages of conducting electronic discussion groups. In particular, he studied the effectiveness of discussions of a sensitive topic amongst 71 Chinese business students. He observed an increased level of participation and interaction amongst participants in the online discussion environment, leading to a higher openness on the part of the students and a higher level of satisfaction with the group discussion experience. It is suggested that online and face-to-face discussion groups occupy different roles within qualitative research (Schneider et al, 2002); online participants contribute shorter comments and are more likely to say only a few words of agreement (Schneider et al, 2002).

Electronic Delphi methods

The Delphi method is designed to foster exploration and distillation of expert opinion (Pike, 2001). While commonly administered by postal means, access to IT makes electronic Delphi methods increasingly attractive. Only a handful of examples exist in the literature. One study investigated the use of computer-related technology (CRT) by counsellors and collected data using a modified futures Internet Delphi method, that comprised a panel of 21 counsellor experts (Cabaniss, 2001).

Electronic opinion polls

Pilot studies are currently assessing the feasibility of allowing voters to vote electronically as part of local and national elections in an attempt to address voter apathy (Gibson et al, 2002; Gwynee, 2001; Reira et al, 2000). Examples from the health field cover the use of computerised opinion polls (Lips, 1998) and interactive conference voting (Goldsmith et al, 1995). However, both focus on obtaining the views of clinicians, as opposed to consumers, and neither evaluate the mode of administration.

Touch screens

Computer-based touch screen systems allow participants to respond to individual questions (or other prompts) by touching the relevant part of a computer screen (Lofland et al, 2000). This method has obvious advantages for users who are less familiar with IT. Many examples of the use of touch screens relate to the administration of questionnaires. Barantiny et al (2000) concluded that touch screen computerised health risk assessments were practical for collecting and monitoring valid cancer risk factor data for hospital outpatients. Lau et al (1996) and Lofland et al (2000) describe the administration and evaluation of the Short-Form 36 (SF-36) via touch screen as routine clinical practice. The latter study compared the costs of touch screen administration with those associated with facsimile and scanning methods, finding them to be comparable, if not more cost-effective, up to an annual survey volume of 1250. Finally, Cooley et al (2001) described an interview data collection system, using a laptop equipped with a touch-sensitive video monitor, to obtain data on sensitive topics, including drug abuse and sexual behaviours associated with HIV and other sexually transmitted diseases.

Example 5: The touch screen questionnaire

In a randomised crossover trial, 149 cancer patients completed the European Organization for Research and Treatment of Cancer Quality of Life Questionnaire-Core 30 (EORTC QLQ-C30), and the Hospital Anxiety and Depression Scale (HADS) on paper and on a touch screen (Velikova et al, 1999). In a further test-retest study 81 patients completed the electronic version of the questionnaires twice, with a time interval of 3 hours between questionnaires. 52 per cent of patients preferred the touch screen to paper, with 24 per cent having no preference. The quality of the data collected with the touch screen system was good, with no missed responses. The authors concluded that computer touch screen quality of life questionnaires were well accepted, with good data quality and reliability.

The strengths and weaknesses of IT methods

Numerous papers document the strengths and weaknesses of replacing traditional research methods with IT equivalents (Thach, 1995; de Leeuw & Nicholls, 1996; Coomber, 1997; Lakeman, 1997; Houston & Fiore, 1998; Mavis & Brocato, 1998; Selwyn & Robson, 1998; Jones & Pitt, 1999; Cook et al, 2000; Fischbacher et al, 2000; Best et al, 2001; Ryan et al, 2002). Most of this literature relates to the use of electronic surveys; however, Lakeman (1997) discusses the benefits and challenges posed by researchers adopting a wider range of Internet methods for data collection. Perhaps one of the most concise critiques of Internet-enabled health surveys, covering various modes of administration (email, Web, newsgroups, etc.), is provided by Fischbacher et al (2000). Jones & Pitt (1999) provide a useful comparison of postal, email and Web methods for health surveys in the workplace. Figure 8.1 summarises the major advantages and disadvantages of replacing traditional research methods with IT-enabled approaches.

	IT Methods	Traditional Methods
Strengths	Cheaper (Foster, 1994; Murray, 1995) Quicker (Houston & Fiore, 1998) No need to take into account time zones (Foster, 1994; Murray, 1995) Removes geographical constraints (Foster, 1994) Easier to recruit hard-to-find target respondents (Tse, 1999) Access to potentially larger sample sizes (Houston & Fiore, 1998) Ease of distribution of questionnaires, etc. (Houston & Fiore, 1998) Reduced chances of coerced participation (Houston & Fiore, 1998) Greater anonymity (Houston & Fiore, 1998) Convenience of time and place of response (Foster, 1994; Houston & Fiore, 1998; Tse, 1999) Faster response times (Mavis & Brocato, 1998) Instant feedback to respondents possible (Foster, 1994) Reduces interviewer effects (Selwyn & Robson, 1998) Reduces time and costs associated with data processing (e.g. transcription) (Foster, 1994; Murray, 1995; Thach, 1995) Improves data integrity, by minimising entry of erroneous or unacceptable data (Houston & Fiore, 1998) Easy transfer of data to other programmes for analysis (Foster, 1994)	Not dependent on respondents' IT skills Assistance available from interviewer (Selwyn & Robson, 1998) Complex instructions and definitions can be given Findings can be validated by observation/non-verbal data (Selwyn & Robson, 1998) Greater richness of data (Selwyn & Robson, 1998)

Figure 8.1 The major strengths and weaknesses of IT and traditional research methods

IT Methods	Traditional Methods
Weaknesses	High set-up costs Increased cost for respondents (Tse, 1999) Time consuming testing and piloting may be required Increased risk of biased samples (Murray, 1995; Houston & Fiore, 1998), including self-selection of participants (Eysenbach & Wyatt, 2002) Excludes certain groups of people who do not have access to IT Problems identifying and circulating to relevant participants (Foster, 1994; Murray, 1995) Problems verifying identities of respondents (Stephenson, 1998) Problems of anonymity of respondents (Murray, 1995) Responses to interview and open-ended questions may not be as in-depth (Murray, 1995) Instructions must be more self-explanatory (Foster, 1994) Lack of visual cues (Mann & Stewart, 2002) Interviewer unable to prompt/probe in a single electronic transaction (Foster, 1994) Problem of entry of inaccurate or malicious data (Murray, 1995) Problems associated with 'netiquette' (Foster, 1994) Assumes reasonable level of IT literacy Lower response rates (Murray, 1995) Less 'rich' data (Selwyn & Robson, 1998) Possible limited generalisability of findings (Eysenbach & Wyatt, 2002)	Requires researchers and participants to be computer literate (Mann & Stewart, 2002) More expensive (Selwyn & Robson, 1998) Sample may be hindered by geographical constraints (Foster, 1994; Murray, 1995) Problems of anonymity (Murray, 1995) Higher risk of problems associated with dominant and shy participants (Selwyn & Robson, 1998) Potential for interviewer bias (Selwyn & Robson, 1998) Data needs to be processed ready for analysis (e.g. interviews transcribed) (Foster, 1994) Increased risk of errors during data processing (Houston & Fiore, 1998)

Figure 8.1 The major strengths and weaknesses of IT and traditional research methods (*continued*)

To summarise then, the major strengths of IT methods are that they are quicker (Houston & Fiore, 1998; Mavis & Brocato, 1998), easier and cheaper (Murray, 1995; Foster, 1994) than paper and telephone counterparts. Mavis & Brocato (1998), found that postal surveys were the most expensive at 92p per reply, compared with 35p for email and 41p for Web surveys. In addition, venue hire, travel and tape recording and transcription costs are reduced (Mann & Stewart, 2002). Administering surveys via the Internet provides access to a rapidly growing and geographically dispersed population of potential participants (Houston & Fiore, 1998). In particular Web-based approaches enable researchers to gain the perspectives of 'hard-to-reach' populations, such as mothers at home with small children, shift workers, people with agoraphobia, housebound people, etc. (Mann & Stewart, 2002). For specific subgroups the Internet may prove a more effective means of gathering data precisely because of the over-representation of particular members of the population. For example, recreational drug users' (Nicholson et al, 1998) and bisexuals (Kaufman et al, 1997) may be particularly elusive for questionnaire or interview but may be amenable to online approaches. Practically, the distribution of questionnaires and interviews electronically is much simpler and easier than paper-based equivalents. It is also suggested that the mechanics of HTML form submission virtually ensure anonymity of participants (Houston & Fiore, 1998), thereby demonstrating the usefulness of electronic methods for collecting data on sensitive topics (Kiesler & Sproull, 1986; Sell, 1997; Joinson, 1999; Joinson, 2001).

Internet-based methods have the added advantage that the researcher does not need to take in to account different time zones (Murray, 1995; Foster, 1994). Participants can respond at a time convenient to them (Foster, 1994; Houston & Fiore, 1998). Several authors note that electronic responses are considerably quicker (Houston & Fiore, 1998; Mavis & Brocato, 1998). Real-time evaluation of incoming data can improve data integrity by ensuring that data are complete and accurate before they are accepted (Houston & Fiore, 1998; Ryan et al, 2002). Utilising IT methods reduces both the time and costs associated with data processing (Foster, 1994; Murray, 1995; Thach, 1995). It had been estimated that up to 20 hours transcription time is needed per hour of interview (Murray, 1995). Electronic interviews remove the need for transcription as the data are already in 'written' form, and readily available for analysis (Murray, 1995). In addition, response collection by means of common gateway interface (CGI) scripts can afford automated data compilation and direct exportation to other software packages (Foster, 1994). In the case of electronic interviews and focus groups, the problem of interviewer effect is reduced (however, the need for reflexivity remains and for discussion on the issues of reflexivity in interviewing see Nicolson's chapter in this volume); such methods also address the problems caused by dominant or shy participants (Selwyn & Robson, 1998). Gunn (2002) contends that, although Web survey design requires ability in programming and Web page design, in preference to knowledge of traditional survey design, technical advantages lie in such effects as the use of frames, differential interfaces for different types of respondent, randomised question sequencing as well as the previously mentioned error checking.

However, these newer approaches suffer from several drawbacks that should be weighed against the perceived benefits before opting for this route. Perhaps the most important weakness, certainly for electronic questionnaires, is the relatively low response rates recorded to date (Kiesler & Sproull, 1986; Murray, 1995; Houston & Fiore, 1998; Mavis & Brocato, 1998; Cook et al, 2000), thus casting doubt on the generalisability of their findings. Cook et al (2000) in a meta-analysis of response rates to Internet surveys identified factors associated with higher response rates including: number of contacts, personalised contacts and pre-contacts. Another major concern with the validity of IT-enabled approaches relates to the exclusivity of contacts with only those who can and do use IT. Published demographics (Kehoe & Pitkow, 1996) show clear inequalities with regard to age (Lakeman, 1997), gender (male rather than female), education (degree-level rather than non-degree educated), ethnicity (European rather than Asian or African) and resources (affluent rather than those with limited financial resources) (Coomber, 1997). However, recent surveys indicate that the user population is becoming more diverse (Houston & Fiore, 1998).

The Internet has certain inherent disadvantages for data collection posed by multiple email addresses, the difficulty in identifying respondents and verifying their identities (Murray, 1995; Stephenson, 1998), and the ease with which data can be submitted (Murray, 1995). Repetitive use of the 'submit' and 'back' buttons on a Web browser allows numerous checked options to be submitted in a fraction of the time required to complete even a single paper-based questionnaire.

The richness of data collected from electronic interactions is not comparable to verbal communication in many ways (Selwyn & Robson, 1998). Computer-mediated communication tends to be a hybrid of oral and written language (Bashier, 1990; Murray, 1995; Selwyn & Robson, 1998) and thus requires different skills from both the researcher and the participant(s). Interviewers are not on hand to prompt or probe interviewees which can, therefore, make it difficult for a good rapport to be established between the interviewer and interviewee. As a result, electronic interviews are generally not as in-depth, or as flexible as face-to-face interviews (Murray, 1995). In addition, a great deal of tacit information is lost as non-verbal data.

New uses of IT to access consumer perspectives

IT offers enormous potential to researchers in accessing the perspectives of those consumers who are frequently overlooked. Examples now evident in the literature include utilisation of bulletin boards (Flaherty, 1995; Nieto, 1996), electronic discussion groups (Hopkins, 2000; Jones & Lewis, 2001) and Internet chat rooms (Woodruff et al, 2001) for research purposes. However, none of these reports specifically targets the views of health consumers.

Flaherty (1995), although not directly discussing research applications, hints at the potential electronic bulletin boards may offer: such systems are versatile, relatively inexpensive, and a practical method for transferring information. An exploratory study, undertaken among gay male bulletin board system users in New York (Nieto, 1996), collected data by means of an electronic questionnaire and structured interview. Jones & Lewis (2001) examined an Internet discussion group for parents of people with Down syndrome and used content analysis to analyse daily discussions over specified periods of time. Similar analyses have examined messages posted to an eating disorder electronic support group (Winzelberg, 1997), and to a Breast Cancer List (Sharf,

1997). Internet chat rooms provide an appealing, convenient and 'naturalistic' environment involving real-time communication (Bailey & Cotlar, 1994). A pilot study indicated that a counsellor-facilitated chat room approach to smoking cessation was both feasible and acceptable among high-risk rural teenager smokers (Woodruff et al, 2001).

A major contribution of the Internet could lie in longitudinal approaches to data collection. 24-hour cable and digital television links to the Internet (Mann & Stewart, 2002) look likely to extend use to communities for whom keyboard and telephone access has previously proved an obstacle, through lack of skills, disability, or cost. More promising, from the researcher's point of view are infra-red keyboards that can be used to send messages via interactive television from a consumer's armchair (Mann & Stewart, 2002). However, data collection must be integrated with other daily activities, e.g. online shopping, contacts with primary health care or social services, recreational activities, such as online bingo, or other forms of interactive cable entertainment.

Finally, more recent IT applications, such as the ever-increasing market for, and sophistication of, mobile telephones, remains unexplored. Mobile telephones can send and receive emails (Alanko et al, 1999) or use wireless application protocol (WAP) to gain access to the Internet using a 'microbrowser' (Mann & Stewart, 2002). Recent developments in speech recognition software have additional potential to involve a greater diversity of people, such as those with visual impairments, learning disabilities, etc.

Many advantages of these newer technologies have been rehearsed earlier in this chapter. Those constrained by face-to-face discussions may be stimulated and less inhibited in a virtual environment (Eley, 1999). Newer approaches are also less costly and generally associated with fewer logistical problems (Woodruff et al, 2001). However each approach has drawbacks, in particular, the ability to access representative samples. Although mobile telephones technically allow text messages to be entered, it is hard to imagine someone participating fully in a virtual focus group by typing out their responses on a 'fiddly' keypad (Mann & Stewart, 2002).

Internet communication is not limited to text (Mann & Stewart, 2002). As the capacity of the Internet increases, voice and video communication become increasingly possible, eliminating the obstacle of the keyboard (Tse, 1999; Mann & Stewart, 2002). According to Mann & Stewart (2002), this will simply get researchers back to where they are now, as there is little substantial difference between voice communication on the Internet and voice telephony. Notwithstanding obvious advantages to video-enhanced communication, such as the reintroduction of visual cues, there are numerous disadvantages, such as technical problems associated with video and transcription time and cost implications (Mann & Stewart, 2002).

The effect of IT on the researcher-consumer relationship

The use of IT to elicit users' views inevitably affects the researcher-consumer relationship. IT methods, possibly with the exception of video-enhanced approaches, share many drawbacks associated with other non-face-to-face qualitative methods, such as telephone interviews (Bashier, 1990). In particular, IT may impact on the power relations between researchers and participants (Denzin & Lincoln, 1994; Sharf, 1999). For example, consumers may feel more empowered and less inhibited to contribute due to the anonymity afforded by IT. However, even online power relations exist (e.g. Kramarae, 1995; Herring, 1996) and it is claimed that researchers (and consumers) find other ways to discriminate between individuals (Mann & Stewart, 2002).

Computer-mediated communication (CMC) is also said to eliminate visual social cues which may inform power relations (Wallace, 1999; refer to Chapters 7 and 11). Matheson (1992) has suggested that working in a medium where social cues are removed increases the focus on other limited cues: email addresses, like postal addresses, carry connotations of culture or status; domain names, such as '.ac' for academic institutions, '.com' for commercial organisations, etc. can give a clue about someone's background (Mann & Stewart, 2002). A lack of facial expressions between the researcher and consumer is likely to have an effect on the data collected, although the use of 'smileys', etc. may help to ameliorate this.

IT-enabled research methods, despite potentially opening wider participation and openness, carry inherent selection biases.

There are many people (e.g. people with a learning disability, people with a visual impairment, etc.) who, for various reasons, either do not have access to IT, or have access, but cannot readily use the technology. Shirley McIver examines such 'hard to reach' groups in more detail in Chapter 10 of this volume and discusses the degree to which such groups can be incorporated into many traditional research methods. In conventional research, participants may, in principle, be drawn from anywhere (although finance, distance and/or language constraints will limit the scope in practice) (Mann & Stewart, 2002). The unrepresentativeness of current Internet access remains the greatest problem for online data collection and potentially limits the generalisability of the findings (Mann & Stewart, 2002; Eysenbach & Wyatt, 2002). In 1998, Loader estimated that only approximately 0.01 per cent of the world's population was online and that this was spread unevenly between countries (Jordan, 1999). Although this figure has increased astronomically over recent years, the vast majority of the world's population have poor, or non-existent, access to the Internet and are, therefore, excluded from attempts to access consumer perspectives. There are significant differences in Internet access both between and within countries, according to age, gender, ethnicity, culture, language, educational status, social class, financial status (Graham & Marvin, 1996), work environments and government regulations (Kendall, 1999). The Internet has predominantly been dominated by young (under 35 years of age) white men (Lockard, 1996; Kendall, 1998; Kendall, 1999), although this trend is beginning to change (Mann & Stewart, 2002). Indeed, evidence suggests that women are generally more interested in health topics and exhibit more active information-seeking behaviour (Fox & Rainie, 2000) and so are more likely to volunteer participation in health questionnaires (Eysenbach & Wyatt, 2002). English is the dominant language on the Internet (Thimbleby, 1998), accounting for about 90 per cent of all interaction. However, this may present a language barrier for many potential users (and researchers) (Mann & Stewart, 2002). Individuals with minimal expertise may feel inhibited, while where people access the Internet (e.g. home, work, cybercafe, etc.) undoubtedly affects individuals' willingness to participate and the responses they give.

Several authors suggest how selection bias might be limited and the representativeness of online samples improved. Fisher et al (1996) and Chappel et al (1999) advocate using clearly defined eligibility criteria, estimating the number of eligible participants from multiple sources, adopting purposive and stratified sampling in order to obtain a representative group, validating email addresses, using screening techniques to improve feedback about where responses originated, and sending reminders to increase the response rate. Potential self-selection bias can be estimated by measuring the response rate, expressed as the number of people completing the questionnaire divided by those who viewed it (Eysenbach & Wyatt, 2002).

Finally, using IT for research purposes has specific ethical implications (Danielson, 1999; Eysenbach & Till, 2001). As Sharf (1999) observes, *it is important to see what is ethically significant about CMC is not the technological change but the social changes it enables* (Sharf, 1999: 70). Although key ethical concerns are common to more traditional research methods, such as privacy, confidentiality and informed consent, newer issues are also emerging. Email can be instantaneously copied or redirected to others, without the writer's knowledge (Sharf, 1999). Individuals responding to online surveys have the option not to reveal their actual names or exact locations, to disguise their identifies, to control how much information they wish to share, etc. (Sharf, 1999). Even self-reported characteristics, such as gender, age, and race as claimed by online participants must be subject to scrutiny (Stone, 1996; Curtis, 1997; Zaleski, 1997). Consequently, attempts have been made to develop principles for fair information exchange on the Internet (Elgesem, 1996). Such principles are embodied within the UK's Data Protection Act, 1998.

Future directions and conclusions

It is safe to predict that the number of people with access to the Internet will continue to grow at a rapid pace (Mann & Stewart, 2002). Diversity of users (and uses) should also increase but usage will likely continue to be concentrated disproportionately among wealthier countries and sections of society (Mann & Stewart, 2002). Although hardware costs have fallen significantly over recent years, infrastructure costs associated with the technology remain and such barriers must be addressed (Mann & Stewart, 2002) before the Internet can truly be regarded as a valuable mechanism. However, the relative exclusivity of Internet use will likely become less of an issue as the technology becomes more widespread and data collection extends to a population more closely representing that reached by established techniques (Houston & Fiore, 1998).

Two facts need to be highlighted when considering the contribution of electronic developments to accessing consumer perspectives. First, the use of IT to conduct research remains largely as 'potential' rather than 'actual'. Those examples that do exist largely originate outside a health research setting (e.g. education ((Thach, 1995; Cook et al, 2000), politics (Fisher et al, 1996), social science (Best et al, 2001; Joinson, 2001), IT (Houston & Fiore, 1998; Ryan et al, 2002), and/or do not relate directly to eliciting users' views. Second, although the Internet partially addresses the perplexing problems of access associated with traditional research methods, its use is still constrained by many threats to validity common to the more established methods; sampling bias (Coomber, 1997), and selection bias (Fischbacher et al, 2000).

A variety of technologies (some yet to be developed) are required to access the widest possible consumer perspectives. Internet communication of the future will involve a hybrid of various forms, with users switching between text, voice, video and graphics, and between synchronous and asynchronous communication (Mann & Stewart, 2002).

To date there is a glaring lack of consultation with users about their preferences for different research methodologies. Mann & Stewart (2002) claim that, from a consumer's perspective, Internet enabled approaches are more participant friendly, are conducive to easy dialogue, allow ideas to be tested in a 'safe environment' and have the potential to extend the research population. However, whether these comments were actually made by consumers or, more likely, were researchers' opinions about what consumers prefer, is unclear. In the absence of other direct evidence one could hypothesise, extrapolated from experience with online pharmacies, that people prefer human interaction to supplement their interface with technology. More research is clearly required on public attitudes to research conducted via the Internet. Any major new technology typically requires that a culture undergoes three predictable stages in adapting to it: substitution, innovation and transformation (Ferguson, 1997). There is little reason to believe that the appearance of lay consumers as active participants in online health care networks will have any different effect on the health care system in following these three stages (Ferguson, 1997). Although participants are generally positive to the use of IT methods, certain sectors of society will always prefer traditional approaches. Instead of completely replacing traditional methods with their IT equivalents, the focus should be on engaging consumers in determining how IT can complement and enhance existing approaches.

References

Alanko, T., Kojo, M., Liljeberg, M. & Raatikainen, K. (1999). Mobile access to the Internet: a mediator-based solution. *Internet Research – Electronic Networking Applications and Policy*, **9**(1), 58–65.

Bailey, E.K. & Cotlar, M. (1994) Teaching via the Internet, *Communication Education*, **43**, 184–193.

Barantiny, G.Y. (2000) Collecting cancer risk factor data from hospital outpatients: use of touch-screen computers, *Cancer Detection and Prevention*, **24**(6), 501–507.

Bashier, R. (1990) Socio-psychological factors in electronic networking, *International Journal of Lifelong Education*, **9**(1), 49–64.

Bell, D.S. & Kahn, C.E. (1996) Health status assessment via the World Wide Web. *Proceedings / AMIA Annual Fall Symposium*, 338–342.

Best, S.J., Krueger, B., Hubbard, C. & Smith, A. (2001) An assessment of the generalisability of internet surveys, *Social Science Computer Review*, **19**(2), 131–145.

Boote, J., Telford, R. & Cooper, C. (2002) Consumer involvement in health research: a review and research agenda. *Health Policy*, **61**, 213–236.

Cabaniss, K. (2001) Counseling and computer technology in the new millennium: an Internet delphi study, *Dissertation Abstracts International Section A: Humanities and Social Sciences*, **62**(1A), 87.

Chappel, D., Fischbacher, C., Richards, R., Oliver, S. & Adshead, F. (1999) Academic training in public health medicine in the UK: findings from an electronic mail census, *Journal of Public Health Medicine*, **21**, 476–479.

Conboy, L., O'Connell, E. & Domar, A. (2001) Women at mid-life: symptoms, attitudes and choices, an Internet based survey, *Maturitas*, **38**(2), 129–136.

Cook, C., Heath, F. & Thompson, R.L. (2000) A meta-analysis of response rates in Web-or internet-based surveys, *Educational and Psychological Measurement*, **60**(6), 821–836.

Cooley, P.C., Rogers, S.M., Turner, C.F., Al-Tayyib, A.A., Willis, G.B. & Ganapathi, L. (2001) Using touch screen audio-CASI to obtain data on sensitive topics, *Computers in Human Behavior*, **17**(3), 285–293.

Coomber, R. (1997) Using the Internet for survey research. *Sociological Research Online*, **2**(2), http://www.socresonline.org.uk/socresonline/2/2/2.html [Accessed 23 April 2003].

Cooper, C. (2000) The use of electronic mail in the research process, *Nurse Researcher*, 7(4), 24–30.

Consumers in NHS Research (2000) *Involving consumers in Research and Development in the NHS: briefing notes for researchers* [online], Hampshire: Consumers in NHS Research Support Unit. http://www.conres.co.uk/pdf/involving_consumers_in_research.pdf [Accessed 7 January 2003].

Curtis, P. (1997). Mudding: social phenomena in text-based virtual realities. In: Kiesler, S., *Culture of the Internet*, Mahwah, NJ: Lawrence Erlbaum Associates, pp. 121–142.

Danielson, P. (1999) Pseudonyms, mailbots, and virtual letterheads: the evolution of computer-mediated ethics. In: Ess, C. (ed.), *Philosophical Perspectives on Computer-Mediated Communication*, Albany: State University of New York Press, pp. 67–93.

Davis, R.N. (1999) Web-based administration or a personality questionnaire: comparison with traditional methods, *Behaviour Research Methods*, **31**, 572–577.

de Leeuw, E. & Nicholls, W.I. (1996) Technological innovations in data collection: acceptance, data quality and costs, *Sociological Research Online*, **1**(4), http://www.socresonline.org.uk/socresonline/1/4/leeuw.html [Accessed 23 April 2003].

Denzin, N. & Lincoln, Y. (1994) *Handbook of qualitative research*, London: Sage Publications.

Edwards, P., Roberts, I., Clarke, M., DiGuiseppi, C., Pratap, S., Wentz, R. & Kwan, I. (2002) Increasing response rates to postal questionnaires: systematic review, *British Medical Journal*, **324**, 1183–1185.

Ehrenberger, H. & Murray, P.J. (1998) Issues in the use of communications technologies in nursing research, *Oncology Nursing Forum*, **25**(10 Suppl), 11–15.

Eley, S. (1999) Nutrition discussion forums: nutrition research using electronic mail, *British Journal of Nutrition*, **81**, 413–414.

Elgesem, D. (1996) Privacy, respect for persons, and risk. In: Ess, C. (ed.), *Philosophical Perspectives on Computer-Mediated Communication*, Albany: State University of New York Press, pp. 45–66.

Eysenbach, G. & Till, J.E. (2001) Ethical issues in qualitative research on internet communities, *British Medical Journal*, **323**(7321), 1103–1105.

Eysenbach, G. & Wyatt, J. (2002) Using the Internet for surveys and health research, *Journal of Medical Internet Research* [online], **4**(2): e13, http://www.jmir.org/2002/2/e13/ [Accessed 23 April 2003].

Ferguson, T. (1997) Health online and the empowered medical consumer, *Journal of Quality Improvement*, **23**(5), 251–257.

Fischbacher, C., Chappel, D., Edwards, R. & Summertown, N. (2000) Health surveys via the Internet: quick and dirty or rapid and robust, *Journal of the Royal Society of Medicine*, **93**, 356–359.

Fisher, B., Margolis, M. & Resnik, D. (1996) Surveying the Internet: democratic theory and civic life in cyberspace, *Southeastern Political Review*, **24**(3), **Pg no ?????**.

Flaherty, R.J. (1995) Electronic bulletin board systems extend the advantages of telemedicine, *Computers in Nursing*, **13**(1), 8–10.

Foster, G. (1994) Fishing the net for research data, *British Journal of Educational Technology*, **25**(2), 91–97.

Fox, S. & Rainie, L. (2000) The online health care revolution: how the Web helps Americans take better care of themselves, Washington: The Pew Internet & American Life Project. http://www.pewinternet.org/reports/toc.asp?Report=26 [Accessed 23 April 2003].

Gibson, R. (2002) Elections online: assessing Internet voting in light of the Arizona democratic primary, *Political Science Quarterly*, **116**(4), 561–583.

Gillespie, G. (1999) But are they satisfied? Technology enables organisations to get faster and more accurate results from patient satisfaction surveys, *Health Data Management*, **7**, 90–92.

Goldsmith, C.H., Duku, E., Brooks, P.M., Boers, M., Tugwell, P.S.L. & Baker, P. (1995) Interactive conference voting. The OMERACT II Committee. Outcome Measures in Rheumatoid Arthritis Clinical Trial Conference, *Journal of Rheumatology*, **22**(7), 1420–1430.

Graham, S. & Marvin, S. (1996) Telecommunications and the city: electronic spaces, urban places, London: Routledge.

Gunn, H. (2002) Web-based surveys: changing the survey process, *First Monday*, **7**(12). http://firstmonday.org/issues/issue7_12/gunn.index.html [Accessed 1 May 2003].

Gwynee, P. (2001) Electronic voting systems make inroads in US local elections – but Internet voting remains a distant prospect, *IEEE Spectrum*, **38**(10), 20–22.

Heerwegh, D. & Loosveldt, G. (2002). Web surveys: the effect of controlling survey access using PIN numbers. Social Science Computer Review **20**(1), 10–21.

Herring, S. (ed.) (1996) Computer-mediated communication: linguistic, social and cross-cultural perspectives, Amsterdam: John Benjamins Publishing.

Hopkins, J. (2000) Could the Internet become a forum for public debate on healthcare quality and funding? *The British Journal of Healthcare Computing & Information Management*, **17**(4), 29–30.

Houston, J.D. & Fiore, D.C. (1998) Online medical surveys: using the Internet as a research tool, *M.D. Computing*, **15**(2), 116–120.

Joinson, A.N. (2001) Knowing me, knowing you: reciprocal self-disclosure in Internet-based surveys, *Cyberpsychology & Behavior*, **4**(5), 587–591.

Joinson, A.N. (1999) Social desirability, anonymity, and Internet-based questionnaires, *Behavior Research Methods, Instruments & Computers*, **31**, 433–438.

Jones, R.S. & Lewis, H. (2001) Debunking the pathological model – functions of an Internet discussion group, *Down Syndrome: Research & Practice*, **6**(3), 123–127.

Jones, R. & Pitt, N. (1999) Health surveys in the workplace: comparison of postal, email and World Wide Web methods, *Occupational Medicine*, **49**, 556–558.

Jordan, T. (1999) Cyberpower: the culture and politics of cyberspace and the Internet, London and New York: Routledge.

Kaufman, J.S., Carlozzi, A.F., Boswell, D.L. & Barnes, L.L.B. (1997) Factors influencing therapist selection among gays, lesbians and bisexuals, *Counselling Psychol Quarterly*, **10**(3), 287–297.

Kehoe, C.M. & Pitkow, J.E. (1996) Surveying the territory: GVU's five WWW user surveys, *World Wide Web Journal*, **1**(3), 77–84.

Kendall, L. (1999) Recontextualising cyberspace: methodological considerations for on-line research. In Jones, S. (ed.), *Doing Internet Research*, Thousand Oaks, CA and London: Sage, pp. 57–75.

Kendall, L. (1998) Meaning and identity in 'Cyberspace': the performance of gender, class and race online, *Symbolic Interaction*, **21**, 129–132.

Kiesler, S. & Sproull, L. (1986) Response effects in the electronic survey, *Public Opinion Quarterly*, **50**, 402–413.

Kim, J., Trace, D., Meyers, K. & Evens, M. (1997) An empirical study of the health status questionnaire system for use in patient-computer interaction, *Proceeding / AMIA Annual Fall Symposium*, **86**, 86–90.

Kramarae, C. (1995) A backstage critique of virtual reality. In: Jones, S. (ed.), *Cybersociety: computer-mediated communication and community*, Thousand Oaks, CA: Sage, pp. 36–56.

Lakeman, R. (2000) Charting the future today: psychiatric and mental health nurses in cyberspace, *Australian & New Zealand Journal of Mental Health Nursing*, **9**, 42–50.

Lakeman, R. (1997) Using the Internet for data collection in nursing research, *Computers in Nursing*, **15**(5), 269–275.

Lau, L.M., Wright, S.O., Garlick-Longhurst, T.J., Graybill, C.S. & Warner, H.R. (1996) Quality assessment and patient participation in care by means of a touch-screen computer, *Clinical Performance & Quality Health Care*, **4**(1), 10–13.

Lips, C.J. (1998) Clinical management of multiple endocrine neoplasia syndromes: results of a computerised opinion poll at the Sixth

International Workshop on Multiple Endocrine Neoplasia and von Hippel-Lindau disease, *Journal of Internal Medicine*, **243**(6), 589–594.

Lipsitz, J.D., Fyer, A.J., Paterniti, A. & Klein, D.F. (2001) Emetophobia: preliminary results of an Internet survey, *Depression and Anxiety*, **14**(2), 149–152.

Loader, B.D. (ed.) (1998) Cyberspace divide: equality, agency and policy in the information society, London and New York: Routledge.

Lockard, J. (1996) Virtual whiteness and narrative diversity. *Undercurrent* [Online], 4, http://darkwing.uoregon.edu/~ucurrent/uc4/4-lockard.html [Accessed 21 September 2001].

Lofland, J.H., Schaffer, M. & Goladfarb, N. (2000) Evaluating health-related quality of life: cost comparison of computerised touch-screen technology and traditional paper systems, *Pharmacotherapy*, **20**(11), 1390–1395.

Mann, C. & Stewart, F. (2002) Internet communication and qualitative research: a handbook for researching online, London: Sage Publications Ltd.

Matheson, K. (1992) Women and computer technology. In: Lea, M. (ed.), *Contexts of computer-mediated communication*, London and New York: Harvester-Wheatsheaf.

Mavis, B.E. & Brocato, J.J. (1998) Postal surveys versus electronic mail surveys. *Evaluation & The Health Professions*, **21**(3), 395–408.

Murray, P.J. (1995) Using the Internet for gathering data and conducting research: faster than the mail, cheaper than the phone, *Computers in Nursing*, **13**(5), 206, 208–209.

Murrelle, L., Bulger, J.D., Ainsworth, B.E., Holliman, S.C. & Bulger, D.W. (1992) Computerised mental health risk appraisal for college students: user acceptability and correlation with standard pencil-and-paper questionnaires, *American Journal of Health Promotion*, **7**(2), 90–92.

Nicholson, T., White, J. & Duncan, D. (1998) Drugnet: a pilot study of adult recreational drug use via the WWW, *Substance Abuse*, **19**, 109–121.

Nieto, D.S. (1996) Who is the male homosexual? A computer-mediated exploratory study of gay male bulletin board system (BBS) users in New York City, *Journal of Homosexuality*, **30**(4), 97–124.

Pike, W. (2001) The HERO e-Delphi system: overview and implementation (draft). http://rhodes.geog.psu.edu/products/Delphi_white_paper.pdf. [Accessed 23 April 2003].

Posavac, E.J., Carey, R.G. & Marin, B.V. (1981) Computers make patient surveys more useful, cost-effective, *Hospitals*, **55**(17), 65.

Reira, A., Rifa, J. & Borrell, J. (2000) Efficient construction of vote tags to allow open objection to the tally in electronic elections, *Information Processing Letters*, **75**(5), 211–215.

Ryan, J.M., Corry, J.R., Atwell, R. & Smithson, M. (2002) A comparison of an electronic version of the SF-36 General Health Questionnaire to the standard paper version, *Quality of Life Research*, **11**(1), 19–26.

Schmidt, W. (1997) World Wide Web survey research: benefits, potential problems and solutions' behaviour, *Behavior Research Methods, Instruments & Computers*, **29**, 274–279.

Schneider, S.J., Kerwin, J., Frechtling, J. & Vivari, B.A. (2002) Characteristics of the discussion in online and face-to-face focus groups, *Social Science Computer Review*, **20**(1), 31–42.

Sell, R.L. (1997) Research and the Internet: an email survey of sexual orientation, *American Journal of Public Health*, **87**(2), 297.

Selwyn, N. & Robson, K. (1998) Using e-mail as a research tool. *Social Research Update* [online] **21**, http://www.soc.surrey.ac.uk/sru/SRU21. html

Sharf, B.F. (1999) Beyond netiquette: the ethics of doing naturalistic discourse research on the Internet. In: Jones, S. (ed.), *Doing Internet Research: Critical Issues and Methods for Examining the Net*, Thousand Oaks: Sage Publications, Inc., pp. 243–256.

Sharf, B.F. (1997) Communicating breast cancer on-line: support and empowerment on the Internet, *Women and Health*, **26**, 65–84.

Stephenson, J. (1998) Patient pretenders weave tangled 'web' of deceit. *JAMA*, **280**(15), 1297.

Stone, A.R. (1996) The war of desire and technology at the close of the mechanical age, Cambridge: MIT Press.

Thach, E. (1995) Using electronic mail to conduct survey research, *Educational Technology*, **March–April**, 27–31.

Thimbleby, H. (1998) Personal boundaries/global stage, *First Monday* [Online], **3**(3), http://www.firstmonday.dk/issues/issue3_3/thimbleby/index.html [Accessed 23 April 2003].

Treadwell, J.R., Soetikno, R.M. & Lenert, L.A. (1999) Feasibility of quality-of-life research on the Internet: a follow-up study, *Quality of Life Research*, **8**, 743–747.

Tse, A.C.B. (1999) Conducting electronic focus group discussions among Chinese respondents, *Journal of the Market Research Society*, **41**(4), 407–415.

Velikova, G., Wright, E.P., Smith, A.B., Cull, A., Gould, A., Forman, D., Perren, T., Stead, M., Brown, J. & Selby, P.J. (1999) Automated collection of quality of life data: a comparison of paper and computer touch screen questionnaires, *Journal of Clinical Oncology*, **17**(3), 998–1007.

Wallace, P. (1999) *The psychology of the Internet*, New York: Cambridge University Press.

Winzelberg, A. (1997) The analysis of an electronic support group for individuals with eating disorders, *Computers in Human Behavior*, **13**, 393–407.

Woodruff, S.I., Edwards, C.C., Conway, T.L. & Elliot, S.P. (2001) Pilot test of an Internet virtual world chat room for rural teen smokers, *Journal of Adolescent Health*, **29**(4), 239–243.

Zaleski, J. (1997) The soul of cyberspace: how new technology is changing our spiritual lives, New York: Harper Collins.

Part Three
Critical Perspectives

9

Users, Research and 'Evidence' in Social Care[1]

Jenny Owen

Introduction

This chapter explores the ways in which policy driven partnerships between health and social care agencies in the UK exploit the views of service users with the aim to improve health and social care delivery. *R&D for a First Class Service* (DoH, 2000) calls for the growth of health research 'communities', including local authority social services departments and voluntary sector organisations and to include health care providers and academic partners. In some areas, local health and social care research and development consortia are now in place, implementing research governance frameworks and providing a base for collaborative projects (Cooke et al, 2002). In addition, much of the current programme of research funded by central government in the UK focuses on areas of joint service provision, including core areas of social work practice. For example, many current research priorities are based on requirements in National Service Frameworks (NSFs) concerning work with older adults, in mental health services and with children's services.[2] There is also considerable emphasis on funding research to support and inform

155

multi-agency services: the Department of Health Service Delivery and Organisation (SDO) R&D funding stream illustrates this, with its orientation towards examining 'whole systems' of care and how they operate (Fulop and Alan, 2000). Last but not least, the 'Consumers in NHS Research' network adopted a new and broader emphasis in spring 2003, when it changed its name to 'INVOLVE: Promoting Public Involvement in NHS, Public Health and Social Care Research' (Consumers in NHS Research Support Unit, 2003).

Emerging research concerning both inter-professional working and inter-agency partnerships in health and social care offers some room for optimism in terms of improved joint service planning and delivery (Hudson, 2000; 2002). However, turning to the specific themes of user perspectives and user-involvement in research, the social care context shows signs of contrasts and tensions with healthcare in some respects, alongside convergence in others. There are contrasts in relation to models of user roles and identities, for example: people accessing social care services have tended to be defined (and sometimes to define themselves) as 'clients', 'service users', 'carers' and occasionally 'citizens' more often than as consumers. A mixed economy of care has been in place in one form or another since the establishment of the welfare state (Cochrane and Clarke, 1993). However at the same time, explicit critiques of consumerism in public services have formed part of most professional and 'user' movement discourses in social care contexts, in response to the quasi-market policies of the 1980s and 1990s. The consumerist emphasis on individual choice and purchaser-provider contracts has been met with a reassertion of notions of citizenship and collective rights, from academic, professional and user vantage points – although the 'consumer' agenda has also been seen as a welcome opportunity to challenge the long-established paternalism in public services (Beresford and Croft, 2001; Barnes, 1999; Barnes, 2002). The term 'service user' has come to be accepted by many in social care as a workable compromise:

> The term 'service user' is problematic, because it conceives of people primarily in terms of their use of services, which may well not be how they would define themselves. However, there is no other umbrella term that can helpfully be used to describe all these overlapping groups. (Beresford and Croft, 2001, 312).

Moving beyond specific phases in welfare regimes and national policies, questions of power, expertise and 'evidence' in social care contexts have come under intense scrutiny at intervals since the 1970s; in parallel, there has been a wide range of practical initiatives in user-involvement in service planning and in research, some predating and some coinciding with those within the NHS (Beresford and Croft, 1987; Barnes, 1997; Consumers in NHS Research Support Unit, 2000). These practical and theoretical interventions challenge some of the dominant premises of current healthcare research, while they complement others. Perspectives from practitioners and researchers are outlined in the first section below, and those led by user initiatives are illustrated in the second section. The chapter concludes with a discussion of some of the choices facing service users and health and social care research communities in the current policy context.

Practitioner and researcher perspectives: is social care research a 'poor relation'?

Social care research as a whole is commonly seen as fragmented, under-resourced and under-utilised: implicitly or explicitly a 'poor relation' vis-à-vis health research in both intellectual and material terms. Certainly, there is a great deal of evidence of a lack of investment and an absence of career structures to support research activity and use in social care, despite a long sequence of government reports pushing for increased research activity and application. The 1980 working party report to the Department of Health and Social Security Research Liaison Group for Local Authority Social Services, 'Directions for Research in Social Work and the Social Services' (DHSS, 1980), for example, identified the need for systematic research in areas such as the specific skills required in different settings, or the implementation of case review systems. A response at the time from a British Association of Social Workers officer made a strong case for researchers

> To engage practitioners in acquiring skills, research skills, even if crude... to inform their role both as practitioners and as social reformers. (Etherington, 1984, 26)

The language of social reform has now given way to more cautious and less overtly political terms: inclusion, effectiveness, partnership, stakeholding. It has been argued that these changes form part of a rise in managerialism which has spanned both Conservative and Labour administrations, actually undermining social care research capacity by shifting resources to performance management instead, despite stated commitments to fostering research (Barnes, 1998). Nevertheless, there is a reminder here that some level of commitment to social change has always been a strong element within social care, coexisting uneasily with elements of social control (Parton, 1999). In terms of resources for social care research in general, many of the debates and concerns have remained remarkably consistent since the 1980s. By 1992, for example, a *Survey of Resources* for personal social services (PSS) research, carried out by the Thomas Coram Research Unit, found that R & D resources were less than 1 per cent of service delivery costs. (quoted in Iwaniec and Pinkerton, 1998, 13). At this stage, over half of all PSS research was being commissioned by the Department of Health, with only 2 per cent resourced directly by local authorities themselves. Iwaniec and Pinkerton noted from the survey that:

> ..*the academic and conceptual framework of social services, and therefore of PSS research, was found to be still underdeveloped. There were no powerful long-established institutions providing leadership... The* British Journal of Social Work *was seldom read by social care workers, and* Community Care, *though widely circulated, gave little space to research findings. However, they found that there was eagerness for sound knowledge to improve practice and to use new validated ideas. (Iwaniec and Pinkerton, 1998, 14)*

In 1994 the DoH published a further report – *A Wider Strategy for Research and Development Relating to Personal Social Services* – which emphasised the need to promote a research culture at all levels. At the time of writing, the recently-established Social Care Institute for Excellence (SCIE) has just commissioned a research review, now recasting the importance of research awareness in terms of post-1997 concerns with public service modernisation:

> *Getting staff to use knowledge derived from research in their day-to-day work is key to the drive to modernise social care. Yet there is a lack of understanding in the field about whether and how staff use the fruits of research. The results... of*

this review of existing research will lay the groundwork for assisting social care organisations to use research evidence in their work. (Social Care Institute for Excellence Media release 25 March 2003)

In this context, two contrasting interventions from professionals and academics continue to influence and shape opportunities for user roles in social care research: the encounter between the 'empirical practice movement' on the one hand, and advocates of 'reflective practice', allied with interpretivist and post-positivist research paradigms, on the other.[3]

The *'empirical practice' movement* has raised a number of fundamental arguments about scope, validity and methods in social care research. Making explicit comparisons with health research models, Sheldon and Macdonald (1999) have argued forcefully for the importance of developing systematic review skills and experimental methods in social care research. They document and seek to challenge the predominance of small-scale, qualitative studies concerning social care:

> *The strictest [research] designs are usually in single figures over a ten year period and are almost always American... The British Journal of Social Work (arguably the premier national journal) has published 356 articles in the last decade. Of these 152 (43%) contain some empirical material, with the majority falling into our 'weak empirical' category, in that they are based on small samples and/or do not adequately address issues of representativeness. This search further revealed only 5 outcome studies, 3 service-effectiveness reviews and no controlled trials. ... When studying the effects of interventions we must learn to live with a hierarchy of research methods and attributive confidence, for only experimental, or at a push, comparative approaches, have the bias-reduction properties to encourage us to head off in one direction rather than another with any sense of security. (Sheldon and Macdonald, 1999, 3).*

The argument here is that the hierarchy of methods which has predominated in much health services research to date should be extended to social care research priorities and practice. This is seen as a move towards remedying the previous lack of capacity, and towards generating appropriate research findings to sustain evidence-based practice; the Centre for Evidence-Based Social Services, based at Exeter University, provides a number of resources and projects to support this (see CEBSS web for some examples, http://www.ex.ac.uk/cebss/). The framework for any joint work would, by implication, emphasise social care practitioners, academics and service users learning from dominant health research models, rather than a more pluralist process of critical exchange and dialogue. A perceived ambivalence towards experimental research methodologies, among social care practitioners, managers and researchers, is still seen as a significant obstacle from this perspective (Macdonald, 2000, 136). Active user involvement in commissioning, designing or conducting research is seen as conditional on particular types of formal training and technical competence, as a CEBSS speaker emphasised at a Consumers in NHS Research conference in 2000:

> *The evidence-based approach... demands that research must meet specific technical requirements.... [the speaker] proposed that users' experience of a service does not qualify them to undertake research – and that they must have the opportunity for proper research training first. (Consumers in NHS Research, 2000b, 38).*

The 'empirical practice' movement has attracted considerable support, for example from the Department of Health in the form of funding for CEBSS. However, it has also been seen as problematic, both from professional and from user perspectives. Firstly, drawing on theories and models of *reflective practice*,[4] social work researchers have argued that the empirical practice movement embodies a simplistic view of what constitutes 'evidence' and of its relationship both with professional practice and with user experience. Webb (2001) provides a thorough overview of the issues at stake here, which have also been explored by Shaw and Shaw (1997) and others (Parton, 1999; Sheppard et al, 2000). Randall (2002) and others have pointed out that this is a new version of an older debate, echoing an exchange first published in social work literature in the late 1970s (see for example Jordan, 1978; Sheldon, 1978).

Webb argues firstly, that the empirical practice movement draws on a positivist epistemological paradigm which has been increasingly contested over the last three decades, and that this movement continues to marginalise interpretive and participatory research traditions (somewhat ironically, since these are gaining increased recognition in health research contexts, as Baxter et al (2001) illustrate). Secondly, he acknowledges that there are both 'hard' and 'soft' versions of the push for evidence-based practice in social care, but that these share a tendency to over-simplify and decontextualise the ways in which people in general (and social care staff and users in particular) make decisions. Here, Webb is neither arguing for an 'anything goes' relativist approach, nor for a refusal to invest in or engage with research processes:

> *More simply, it is claimed that social work simply does not and cannot work in the way evidence-based practice suggests. Research shows that heuristics play a much more decisive role, even in the face of evidence, than the evidential approach allows for. This suggests that social work requires a model which is much more nuanced and sensitive to local and contextual factors. That is, a model which recognises, in line with research in connectionist and network analysis, that social actors operate with a limited rationality due to the indeterminacy, uncertainty and spontaneous effects of networked systems which change over time. (Webb, 2001, 76).*

Webb's argument, then, is for a critical approach to developing research capacity, to considering methodological options and to situating research processes within an understanding of professional values and organisational practices. In contrast with Sheldon and Macdonald (1999), the degree of discretion and autonomy associated with social work (and other professional roles) is seen here as a positive resource for dialogue and reflection, rather than as an obstacle to change. This has clear parallels with current research perspectives in primary health care (Cooke et al, 2002); it is also consistent with the approach recently adopted by the Social Care Institute of Excellence (SCIE) following a stakeholder consultation exercise with services users, practitioners and academics, and with recent statements from the Social Services Inspectorate (SSI). SCIE now has a stated commitment to seeing 'all sources of knowledge come equally to the table', whether derived from user and carer experience, practitioner experience and knowledge, examples of practice innovation, evaluations or qualitative and quantitative research. The task of devising a methodology for reviewing and synthesising knowledge from these diverse sources is acknowledged to be challenging (Edwards, 2002, 15). On a related tack, the Social Services Inspectorate's annual report in 2002–3 noted that

> *The evidence shows that the services which are most effective, are those where frontline social workers are supported in a clear managerial framework and where they are encouraged to develop 'reflective practice', improving their professional skill in making judgements in very complex situations. The Victoria*

Climbié Inquiry Report notes that 'practice should be governed by professional judgement not by rules and procedures' (p. 357). (SSI Annual Report, 2002–2003, emphasis in original).

An overview of themes concerning reflective practice, research and user-involvement was provided by a seminar series funded by the Economic and Social Research Council in 1999–2000, 'Theorising Social Work Research (National Institute for Social Work, 2000: ESRC-funded seminar series 'Theorising Social Work Research'.[5] This has articulated a broad approach, explicitly encouraging collaboration rather than competition between academic centres with differing emphases and perspectives. The draft strategic framework produced from the seminar series in March 2000 acknowledged the small and fragmented academic base for social work and social care research, but also pointed to examples of theoretical and empirical achievement, particularly in relation to user-involvement:

> *Because social work has not been recognised in disciplinary terms in many parts of the academy, and because of a characteristic humility in presentation and lack of theoretical bite, social work's track record ... often remains unacknowledged. We therefore watch other disciplines promoting theoretical knowledge for involving users... for instance, in the sure and certain knowledge that we have a twenty year history in this aspect on which we have not sufficiently capitalised.*
> *(http://www.nisw.org.uk/strategicframework.html accessed 1/10/00).*

Both the draft strategic framework and specific seminar papers went to identify the nature of the relationship between service users' movements and the social work research community as the key priority to continue to address in theoretical and empirical studies. More recently, the 'Making Research Count' network[6] has begun to propose and operationalise the notion of 'knowledge-based practice'; this is consistent with the recent SCIE statements noted above, since it 'conceives of a triangle of research, practitioner wisdom and service user perspectives underpinning the development of practice in social work and social care' (Humphreys et al, 2003, 41). This is a clear move in the direction of continuing broad critical exchange and dialogue, including user expertise, rather than uncritically adopting dominant health research models of evidence-based practice.

To summarise then: contrasting academic and professional perspectives on social care research share a concern with the uneven and under-resourced nature of research capacity and infrastructure in social care. Currently, research funding is supporting a wide range of initiatives in research development and dissemination; although there is consensus about the need to support and invest in social care research, there are some substantial differences of opinion about appropriate principles and practices. We now turn to the ways in which some of these differences have been addressed from service user perspectives.

User-led perspectives and initiatives: redefining the terms?

To different degrees, both the empirical practice movement and the reflective practice perspective can be seen as problematic from user standpoints. The former adheres to an epistemological framework and a hierarchy of research methods which user movements have challenged over two decades as marginalising their expertise (Gibbs, 1999); the emphasis is much more on the perceived quality of the research 'product' than the process. The latter recognises a more complex relationship between 'product' and 'process', and allows much more scope for dialogue, partnership and acknowledgement of power relationships between researcher, service user and research 'subject'; nevertheless, the terms of engagement remain substantially defined by academics and professionals (Barnes, 2002). Examples of interventions and challenges which draw directly on user experience and self-organisation in social care contexts include some from user networks and some from academics working in close collaboration with user networks. Many refer to some form of continuum in the degree of control exercised by user and/or researcher in the research process, from 'professional exclusive' at one end to 'lay exclusive' at the other (Baxter et al, 2001, 48–53).[7] (See also Chapter 10 in this volume).

To take an initial example which has focused strongly on combining theoretical commentaries with practical initiatives, Peter Beresford and Suzy Croft have set out to integrate their combined experience in using, delivering and researching social care services, in a series of publications dating from the 1980s. Beresford is now Professor of Social Policy and Director of the Centre for Citizen Participation at Brunel University, as well as a participant in the psychiatric system survivors' movement; Croft is a senior social worker in palliative care, a practice teacher and a research fellow at Brunel. Both are involved in the Shaping Our Lives user-controlled development network[8] (see http://www.shapingourlives.org.uk/network.htm).

Early papers articulated the ways in which service users have commonly been excluded both from service planning and from research processes in social care; later commentaries identified forms of user experience of research characterised by 'extraction' (data gathering) and then 'consultation fatigue' (Beresford and Croft, 2001, 296). More recent analyses have explored the implications of emerging 'user-involvement' initiatives within wider New Labour social policy developments, arguing that welfare system user movements have now begun to redefine the boundaries with respect to research:

> *Service user campaigners aren't just calling for social policy to ask for and include their views. Researchers have been doing this for years – surveying service users, then analysing, interpreting and acting upon them as they see fit. Service users are demanding that social policy goes beyond seeing them as a data source... [they] can and want to offer their own analyses, interpretations and plans for action... Service users are now calling into question the legitimacy of traditional research. (Beresford, 2001, 508)*

The Shaping Our Lives network has produced a user-led examination of how 'outcomes' are understood in social care (Turner, 1998); this has laid the basis for four further development projects, each located with a local user network, and addressing the specific views of older people, disabled groups in ethnic minority communities, mental health service users and Black communities.[9] These are examples in which the initiative is firmly with user organisations rather than academic centres or professionals, and which address the ways in which outcomes are conceptualised as well as the details of particular services or user experiences. The 1998 report, for example, emphasised users' concern to ensure that research examines 'process' as well as 'outcome': 'positive outcomes cannot come without good pro-

cesses' (Turner, 1998, 16). While the empirical practice movement emphasises training of users *by* researchers – as indicated
above – the Shaping Our Lives initiatives propose *mutual* learning processes, drawing on the expertise of all parties in a
research or evaluation project.

A second set of examples comes from one of the 'new social
movements' which have challenged paternalistic approaches to
welfare since the 1970s: most prominently the women's and gay
movements, networks of people with disabilities and black and
minority ethnic groups.[10] Networks of people with disabilities, for
example, have played a substantial part in questioning established
research processes and paradigms. Gibbs (1999) provides a
cogent overview, drawing particularly on work done at the
Derbyshire Centre for Inclusive Living (DCIL), in his contribution to the ESRC 'Theorising Social Work Research' seminar
series. He argues that relations between disabled people and the
research community have moved from 'abrasion' through 'assertion' to 'convergence', to a point at which 'co-production' can be
envisaged in some circumstances (Gibbs, 1999). The development
of the social model of disability at a theoretical level has gone
hand in hand with the development of new forms of professional
and user practice. User control of support packages is an example
of user-controlled service provision, when disabled people use
the Direct Payments system to employ carers themselves, rather
than depending on predefined packages of care. In research contexts, initiatives to ensure that funding bodies adopt clear criteria
concerning access and involvement for users with disabilities characterised the 'assertion' stage in the mid-1990s. However, it is
important to keep in focus just how 'abrasive' some of the early
encounters between researchers and disabled people were; Gibbs
gives the example of a 1972 study of residential institutions
(Miller and Gwynne, 1972, and subsequent critique in Hunt,
1981):

> *Even while fully recognising the 'living death' and 'inherent pathogenic char-*
> *acteristics' of institutional living, the researchers made no reference to com-*
> *munity alternatives or recommendations for fundamental change, but*
> *concluded that 'the essential task to be carried out is to help the inmates to*
> *make the transition from social death to physical death…' The depth of*
> *feeling this research experience generated is undiminished to this day. (Gibbs,*
> *1999, 2)*

Gibbs gives more recent examples of studies which disabled user networks have experienced as 'purpose co-working' with researchers – the 'convergence' model – generating insights which user organisations can use to critique and develop their own strategies and practices; Priestley's study (1999) for example provided findings on the ways in which 'integrated living' models initiated by disabled networks interfaced with community care legislation, informing continued discussion and policy development within those networks. Finally, Gibbs emphasises that controversy continues about the potential of user-led research approaches (see for example the critique from Oliver, 1997, reflecting pessimistically on his own experience as activist and researcher in disabilities studies).

Thirdly, the broader theoretical and the policy implications of changing forms of user involvement in health and social care settings have been explored by a number of observers: Harrison and Mort (1998), for example, found evidence of health policymakers and managers 'playing the user card' to legitimise their own decisions, although findings from later studies include evidence of significant lay challenges both to managerial and to medical power (Milewa et al, 2002). With reference to social care, Marian Barnes provides a particularly strong theoretical overview (Barnes, 2002), drawing on over a decade of close collaboration with user organisations. Making the link with long-established feminist work on 'standpoint-specific' knowledge, Barnes emphasises the ways in which user movements – along with other marginalised social groups – 'offer a critique of the rational scientific basis of knowledge production. They expose the particularity of the standpoint from which knowledge is produced' (Barnes, 2002, 322). Exploring areas rather glossed over by the pluralistic SCIE approach noted above, Barnes emphasises that user and professional perspectives will not be able to 'come equally to the table' without radical changes, both in organisations and in research processes:

> *We need a practice of deliberation which explicitly recognises and encompasses inequalities of power and diversity of experience and expression, rather than assuming that such inequality and diversity will be accommodated within processes governed by universalist notions of fairness and competence...Disabled people's movements and survivor movements are experiencing dilemmas encountered by other social movements, not least the women's movement, in occupying spaces for deliberation that have opened up, without succumbing to*

co-option – to adopting official rules rather than transforming the rules by which the game is played. (Barnes, op. cit., 324 and 329).

Barnes' work draws on social theory more thoroughly and more explicitly than many other contributors to recent user-involvement initiatives, and on debates arising from Habermas' work on communicative competence in particular. Significantly, her emphasis on the need to 'transform the rules' extends to 'exploring and taking on board the emotional, expressive and embodied aspects of experience as well as its rational cognitive aspects' (2002, 330). One of the implications of this, for researchers and for practitioners, is that messages will not always be communicated in familiar, comfortable or conventionally-accepted terms; consensus will not always be possible. Barnes describes, for example, an encounter between users who described the psychiatric system as abusing their rights, and a psychiatrist who responded defensively that they needed to 'understand the system' more fully before judging it. (Barnes, 2002, 329).

Alongside its investment in exploring how health-related models of research and evidence-based practice might apply in social care, the Department of Health has also funded scoping studies of user-involvement in research in settings outside the NHS. In 2001, the 'empowerment sub-group' of the Consumers in NHS Research advisory group published a very comprehensive overview: *Small Voices, Big Noises – Lay Involvement in Health Research: Lessons from Other Fields* (Baxter et al, 2001). The research team worked in collaboration with 'Folk.us', the Forum for Collaboration with Users in Research based in the Psychology Department at Exeter University, and also received some funding via CEBSS. Sources and examples used in the study included participatory research approaches in developing countries, community development projects in the UK and user-led initiatives in social care – with the latter acknowledged to be at the leading edge in terms of involving users (Baxter et al, 2001, 81). The resulting report combines accessible language and presentation, practical case-study examples and proposed typologies of user-involvement; the report also places its examples in the context of current debates about knowledge, evidence and practice, adopting a broad definition of research (Baxter et al, op. cit., 71–2).

Barriers and factors identified as facilitating user-involvement are usefully broken down into those associated with people (e.g. values, attitudes); those concerning process (e.g. timing of user participation), and those concerning resources (e.g. how far the time needed to foster sustained user participation is catered for within project funding). There are clear and explicit examples of collaborative approaches; chapter five, for example, itemises examples of skills and knowledge which users may need to access, about research techniques, alongside those which researchers may need to access about each specific lay context. As suggested above in connection with the Shaping Our Lives initiatives, the impetus here is for partnership, rather than for users to 'catch up with' researchers. The report stresses the value of relatively small-scale studies, with a clear focus on contributing to improving services and/or tackling perceived problems. The broad conclusion from the study is that:

> *Overall, ideas and methods for active lay involvement from other fields are practical and applicable to health research. (Baxter et al, 2001, viii)*

However, the study also picks up the same elements of tension between evidence based practice models and broader approaches to research which were noted above:

> *The discussion leaves us with some questions about the way in which 'evidence-based practice' now equates to 'good practice' in the fields of health and social care. Frequently 'evidence' is narrowly interpreted only as 'scientific'. But there are other sorts of evidence, equally valid, that can be acquired by using different approaches to research and enquiry. (Gomm and Davies, 2000; cited in Baxter et al, 2001, 70)*

To summarise then, a relatively long track record in exploring the user-researcher relationship in social care means that a diverse range of coinciding models, initiatives and theoretical interventions are now being consolidated and disseminated. Concern to avoid a narrow definition of research and of evidence-based practice is shared by many user networks, practitioners and researchers; in this sense, the social care context still differs significantly from most NHS research settings. Some of the differences are yet to be explored fully, although continuing policy developments will eventually provoke further clarification. In the next section of this chapter, I move on to consider some of the 'crunch points' at which this is likely to take place.

Choices, questions, challenges

The Labour government's 'modernisation' impetus in public services has reconfigured many of the arenas in which users, researchers and practitioners address inter-relationships between research, policy and practice. As Marian Barnes argues, some new spaces for intervention have emerged, but they certainly do not resemble the proverbial level playing-field; many user networks and social care researchers would also argue that the boundaries and the goal posts have yet to reach steady positions. New organisations such as SCIE, for example, have adopted a relatively broad approach to research and expertise; I have argued above that this is more compatible with user-led perspectives in research than the 'evidence-based practice' model and the associated hierarchy of research methods which have been dominant for many years in health research contexts. The SCIE approach also helps to challenge the 'poor relation' status which has sometimes been attached to social care research, and to recognise expertise within both user and practitioner networks. On the other hand, there is a continuing government preoccupation with evaluating 'what works' and with setting crudely-defined targets to be met in relatively short timescales; this has attracted increasing levels of concern, both because it has sometimes blurred the boundaries between performance management, research and evaluation (Biott and Cook, 1999; Talbot, 2000), and because the pace and top-down character of many policy developments can marginalise user participation in particular, as well as dialogue or reflection in a more general sense (Baxter et al, 2001).

In concluding this chapter, I want to note two specific areas in which we can expect some of the tensions between user-involvement models in social care and those in health to crystallise. This may help to produce new resolutions, on a basis of partnership; alternatively, it may embed some particular perspectives at the expense of others. Two key areas to consider in this respect concern developments in frameworks for research ethics and governance, and avenues for research funding and dissemination.

Firstly, the *research governance framework (RGF)* recently developed by the Department of Health aims to raise standards and to clarify the responsibilities of different parties in the research process; it addresses the domains of ethics, 'scientific rigour', access to findings, health and safety and financial probity. A baseline assessment exercise for RGF in social care (DoH, 2003a) found that many SSDs were not ready to implement the RGF in its current form; 85 per cent of authorities had less than half the necessary systems in place to implement it. No authority was fully ready to comply. Only 14 per cent of authorities said they had systems in place to give ethical approval to research, and only 8 per cent had an established peer review process.

Proposals have also been developed for joint health and social care consideration of frameworks for research ethics and governance (see DoH, 2003b). Will this lead to a reconsideration of needs and structures across the whole range of health research and social research? Or will there be pressure to adapt existing NHS research ethics structures to social care domains? Existing NHS Research Ethics Committees have been criticised for over-representing large-scale, experimental studies, medicalised approaches to health and a 'gate-keeping' role rather than a facilitative one (Lewis, 2002); in all these respects, they pose significant problems for user-involvement in research. Lewis and others have identified some fundamental questions to address, in attempting to arrive at joint health and social care approaches to research ethics. Some of these echo and reinforce points made earlier.

Firstly, Lewis notes some important organisational contrasts between the NHS and social care contexts: for example, few areas of social research or social care research actually depend on social care organisations for access to subjects, whereas NHS Trusts and other organisations are the main channel of access for health service researchers, both to populations and to medical records. Simply extending NHS research ethics committee structures (RECs) to social care organisations would still leave vast areas of potentially sensitive social research untouched: research on prisons, asylum seeking, school refusal or policing are examples. Secondly, Lewis emphasises that major ethical questions tend to

arise *during* a social research process more often than at the
design stage: balancing the need for confidentiality against the
need for effective child protection, for example, in research with
looked-after children. Here, Lewis argues that the need is for
advice to support researchers in making appropriate judgements
– something not currently within the scope of RECs, with their
gatekeeping and approval-providing (or withholding) roles.

Lewis also moves beyond these practical considerations to illustrate the ways in which 'ethics committees treat vulnerability as
the defining characteristic of the human condition', focusing
increasingly on risk management and avoiding litigation (Furedi,
2002, quoted in Lewis, 2002, 5). Lewis rejects this model, challenging its implicit paternalism and arguing for the individual
user's right and ability to make an informed decision to participate in a research process. Her concluding proposal is for the
Academy of the Learned Societies for the Social Sciences to
develop consensus about good practice and to provide expert
advice to researchers (whether from academic, practitioner or
user backgrounds), across the whole range of social science and
social care research. At the time of writing, then, there is still a
significant gap between the more facilitative approach characteristic of social care contributors to debates on ethics and governance, and the 'gatekeeping' emphasis which remains more
characteristic of NHS and Department of Health proposals.
Arguably, it is the former which offers greater scope and recognition for lay participation; the evolving policy developments concerning ethics and governance in research will clearly affect scope
for lay involvement. In service planning contexts, recent consultations continue to emphasise users' interests in extending social
care models to health contexts – as reiterated at a King's Fund
workshop in 2002, for instance:

> *Participants commented that social services had good ways of involving service
> users in budget meetings and joint investment programme planning. Social ser-
> vices had also introduced mechanisms to give service users more direct control
> over their services through direct payment schemes. The group felt that the NHS
> needed to learn from this, and, where possible, share structures which social ser-
> vices had established rather than setting up separate ones for the NHS. There
> were also fears that social approaches to health, focusing on the health and
> social needs of the individual, might be lost in favour of a more medicalised
> approach to health. (King's Fund, 2002, 6).*

It remains to be seen whether or not this perspective will be extended to research contexts, both in terms of ethics and governance and in other respects.

Research funding and dissemination processes are the second area in which differing perspectives from health and social contexts are apparent. Reports such as the one from Baxter et al (2001) on user-involvement in research in social care and community contexts have emphasised the particular importance of relatively small-scale studies, often primarily qualitative, which address potential areas of change and which can accommodate flexible forms of collaboration. Here, the emphasis may be on a realist epistemological framework (Pawson and Tilley, 1997), theorising processes of change and offering scope for transferability; or it may be on problem solving, action research and empowerment at a local level. Neither of these approximates to the 'generalisability' usually regarded as a defining requirement for health research, and consistently emphasised both within the 'evidence-based practice' movement and in Department of Health research programmes. This takes us back to the heart of the argument about a hierarchy of methods: these are precisely the kinds of studies which Sheldon and others have argued are already over-represented in social care research (Sheldon and Macdonald, 1999). For the moment, the Department of Health funds initiatives right across the spectrum of paradigms and methods: advocates for extending the use of experimental research designs in social care coexist with advocates for a broad definition of research and for 'knowledge-based' practice which encompasses user voices. The latter may still be in the minority in terms of sheer funding volume, but their visibility is increasing. Research programmes in the Department of Health, the Joseph Rowntree Foundation and some other organisations now require that proposals should at least address the question of user-involvement explicitly, although this is not closely monitored once projects are launched, which is a potential weak point. In social care, some dialogue has been initiated concerning peer-reviewed publications: Beresford et al (2001), for example, have suggested some specific criteria for peer-reviewed journals to consider in order to bring user voices into the mainstream; these include accessibility of published formats, acknowledgement of user authorship and collaboration, recognition of user-led discourses and inclusion of user perspectives in production and decision-making processes (in research as well as in service delivery).

Much research effort continues to be shaped and governed by the reward structures and performance management systems which prevail in higher education: in particular the Research Assessment Exercise which takes place periodically. It remains the case that conventional, single-authored books and articles attract more recognition than the relatively time-consuming and often smaller-scale collaborative partnerships which are acknowledged to facilitate user-involvement. In principle, it would be quite feasible to alter this emphasis, and for example to build in specific research assessment criteria which recognise and reward partnership working between user networks and university departments. This would be a logical way to build on the ground already covered by the scoping studies and the guidelines for promoting user-involvement such as those produced by the Department of Health (Consumers in NHS Research, 2000). Without changes of this kind, it is hard to envisage a sustained shift towards 'co-production' between users, practitioners and academics in research processes.

Conclusion

Discourses which once characterised only radical user networks have certainly migrated into parts of mainstream policy and research communities in recent years: 'nothing about us without us' for example, a slogan originating from networks of people with disabilities later appeared as an unremarkable heading in the King's Fund report cited above (King's Fund, 2002). Other terms have not migrated so readily. Social care literature, for example, features regular references to 'survivors' (in the mental health system, in child abuse or domestic violence situations) and to debates about 'anti-oppressive practice'; these are clear references to the importance of unequal power relations, in families, in communities and in service or research contexts. Healthcare professionals and researchers may talk about 'cancer survivors', but the emphasis here is on the condition, not the context. Most remain more at ease with a blander vocabulary, in which for the moment 'users', 'consumers', 'patients' and 'stakeholders' all coexist; there continue to be diverging assumptions about the range of roles and statuses these terms suggest.

The current policy impetus for increased collaboration across health and social care boundaries is unfolding in a pluralistic context, concerning paradigms, methods and values in research. Assumptions which have been taken for granted in the past – hierarchies of methods, for example, or a passive role for service users – have been eroded both by government policy and by independent user or community initiatives. In this climate, there is genuine scope for user-involvement models and initiatives from social care contexts to inform health research theory and practice. As to how far this will be achieved in practice, the jury is still out; however, developments concerning research ethics and governance on the one hand, and funding and dissemination on the other, offer clear opportunities to reach a judgement.

Notes

1. In this chapter, I am using the term 'social care' in the broad sense, to refer to 'the entire spectrum of welfare provision within the personal social services *including* social work' (Macdonald, 2000, 117).

2. National Service Frameworks (NSFs) are one of the current government's measures designed to improve service quality and provision in the UK. They 'set national standards and identify key interventions for a defined service or care group; put in place strategies to support implementation; establish ways to ensure progress within an agreed time-scale' (taken from the Department of Health web page on NSFs, http://www.doh.gov.uk/nsf/index.htm).

3. There is not enough space here to do justice to the full range of debates concerning 'ways of knowing' in health and social care research, and there is a danger of using 'positivism' as the 'convenient term of abuse' referred to by Shaw (1999) and others. The contrast I am referring to here, very briefly, is between a positivist tradition on the one hand, and a wide range of interpretivist and realist, post-positivist traditions on the other. The former tradition 'argues that knowledge about the world can only be gained through accumulating facts that have been discovered through controlled, replicable and objective observation or experiment' (Brechin and Sidell, 2000, 11); the emphasis is on arriving at generalisable findings, laws and causal explanations. The latter traditions all argue that the relationship between theory, observation and interpretation is more complex than implied by positivism, particularly

(though not solely) in the social world. So the emphasis here is on theorising patterns rather than laws, on research as embodying processes of interpretation rather than neutral observation, and on presenting findings which are 'transferable' between specific contexts rather than universally generalisable. For a more subtle and detailed discussion of all these points, see for example Shaw (1999), chapter three; Silverman (1993), chapter two; Pawson and Tilley (1997), chapters one and nine; Williams (2000). Brechin and Sidell (op.cit) make the links between the general arguments and research processes in health and social care contexts.

4. 'Reflective practice is more than just thoughtful practice. It is the process of turning thoughtful practice into a potential learning situation ... Reflective practice entails the synthesis of self-awareness, reflection and critical thinking' (Eby, 2000, 52).

5. see http://www.elsc.org.uk/socialcareresource/tswr/tswrindex.htm

6. Making Research Count' is a collaborative venture between seven English universities, a number of Local Authority Social Services Departments and (in some areas) NHS and voluntary organisations. (Humphreys et al, 2003).

7. This report provides a useful and detailed illustration of this spectrum, addressing both the quality and the level of user participation.

8. Shaping Our Lives is a UK national user-controlled development project and network, set up in 1996 with initial funding from the Department of Health; subsequently it has received funding from the Joseph Rowntree Foundation. It has also established a National User Group to develop thinking on service provision and outcomes from a user perspective. (Beresford et al, 2001).

9. http://www.shapingourlives.org.uk/development.htm

10. For a full discussion of new social movements, user participation and citizenship, see for example Fiona Williams (2000) and Barnes (1999). Both address the difference between movements or networks based on identity and those based on interests.

References

Barnes, M. (1997) *Care, Communities and Citizens.*

Barnes, M. (1998) Editorial, *Social Services Research*, 4, i–ii.

Barnes, M. (1999) 'Users as citizens: collective action and the local governance of welfare', *Social Policy & Administration*, 33: 1, pp. 73–90.

Barnes, M. (2002) 'Bringing difference into deliberation? Disabled people, survivors and local governance', *Policy & Politics*, 30: 3, pp. 319–331.

Baxter, L., Thorne, L. and Mitchell, A. (2001) *Small Voices, Big Noises – Lay Involvement in Health Research: Lessons from Other Fields*, Exeter: Consumers in NHS Research.

Beresford, P. (2001) 'Service Users, Social Policy and the Future of Welfare', *Critical Social Policy*, 21: 4, pp. 494–512.

Beresford, P. and Croft, S. (1987) 'Are we really listening? "The Client Speaks" by John Meyer and Noel Timms' in T. Philpot (ed.) *On Second Thoughts: Reassessments of the Literature of Social Work*, Surrey: Reed Business Publishing/Community Care.

Beresford, P. and Croft, S. (2001) 'Service Users' Knowledges and the Social Construction of Social Work', *Journal of Social Work*, 1: 3, pp. 295–316.

Beresford, P., Brough, P. and Turner, M. (2001) 'Where Do You Stand with Service Users?' *Journal of Social Work*, 1: 1, pp. 119–120.

Biott, C. and Cook, T. (2001) Local Evaluation of a national pilot pro- gramme: integrating performance management and participatory eval- uation, *Evaluation*, 6: 4 pp. 399–413.

Brechin, A. and Siddell, M. (2000) 'Ways of knowing', in R. Gomm and C. Davies (eds) *Using Evidence in Health and Social Care*, London: Sage/Open University.

Cochrane, A. and Clarke, J. (1993) *Comparing Welfare States: Britain in International Context*, London: Sage.

Consumers in NHS Research Support Unit (2000a) *Involving Consumers in Research and Development in the NHS: Briefing Notes for Researchers*, Winchester: the Help for Health Trust.

Consumers in NHS Research (2000b) *Research: Who's Learning?* Report of the conference held in January 2000 at Kensington Town Hall, London, p. 38.

Consumers in NHS Research Support Unit (2003) *News*, Spring 2003.

Cooke, J.M., Owen, J. and Wilson, A. (2002) 'Research and Development at the Health and Social Care Interface in Primary Care: a Scoping Exercise in one National Health Service Region', *Health and Social Care in the Community*, 10: 6, pp. 435–444.

DHSS (1980) 'Directions for Research in Social Work and the Social Services, 1980. A working party report to the DHSS Research Liaison Group for Local Authority Social Services', *British Journal of Social Work*, 10, pp. 207–217.

Department of Health (1990) *Taking Research Seriously*, London: HMSO.

Department of Health (1994) A Wider Strategy for Research and Development Relating to Personal Social Services London: HMSO.

Department of Health (1998) Modernising Social Services: Promoting Independence, Improving Protection, Raising Standards. London: The Stationery Office.

Department of Health (2000) *Research and Development for a First Class Service*, Department of Health; Leeds.

Department of Health (2001) *Research Governance Framework for Health & Social Care* . London: Department of Health.

Department of Health (2003a) Research Governance in Social Care: The findings of the 2002 baseline assessment exercise at http://www. doh.gov.uk/research/documents/BAreport.PDF

Department of Health (2003b). Progress With the Implementation of the Research Governance Framework in the Field of Social Care http://www.doh.gov.uk/research/rd1/researchgovernance/socialcarepro-gressreport.htm

Eby, M. (2000) 'Understanding professional development', in Brechin et al (eds) *Critical Practice in Health and Social Care*, London: Sage/Open University.

Edwards, A. (2002) 'What is "Knowledge" in Social Care?' *MCC: Building Knowledge for Integrated Care*, 10: 1, pp. 13–16.

Etherington, S. (1984) 'Social research and social work practice', *Research, Policy and Planning*, 2: 1, pp. 25–27.

Fulop, N. and Allen, P. (2000) National Listening Exercise: Report of the Findings. http://www.sdo.lshtm.ac.uk/PDF/ListeningExerciseReport.pdf

Furedi, F. (2002) 'Don't rock the research boat', *Times Higher Education Supplement*, January 11, p. 20.

Gibbs, D. (1999) 'Disabled People and the Research Community', paper presented to the ESRC Seminar Series 'Theorising Social Work Research: Who Owns the Research Process?' Belfast, 20.9.99. Available electronically at http://www.elsc.org.uk.socialcareresource/tswr/seminar2/gibbs.htm

Gomm, R. and Davies, C. (2000) *Using Evidence in Health and Social Care*, London: Sage.

Harrison, S. and Mort, M. (1998) 'Which champions, which people? Public and user involvement in health care as a technology of legitimation', *Social Policy & Administration*, 32: 1, pp. 60–70.

Hudson, B. (2000) 'Social Services and Primary Care Groups: a window of collaborative opportunity?' *Health and Social Care in the Community*, 8: 4, pp. 242–50.

Hudson, B. (2002) 'Interprofessionality in health and social care: the Achilles' heel of partnership?' *Journal of Interprofessional Care*, 16: 1, pp. 7–17.

Humphreys, C., Berridge, D., Butler, I. and Ruddick, R. (2003) 'Making Research Count: the Development of 'Knowledge-Based Practice', *Research, Policy and Planning*, 21: 1, pp. 41–49.

Hunt, P. (1981), Settling accounts with the parasite people: a critique of 'A Life Apart' by E.J. Miller and G.V. Gwynne. Disability Challenge, 1: 37–50.

Iwaniec, D. and Pinkerton, J. (1998) Making Research Work: Promoting Child Care Policy and Practice, Chichester: Wiley.

Jordan, B. (1978) 'A Comment on "Theory and Practice in Social Work"', *British Journal of Social Work*, 8: 11, pp. 23–25.

King's Fund (2002) *Shaping Our Lives – Patient and Public Involvement in Health: the Views of Health and Social Care Users*. Report from the workshop held at the King's Fund in April 2002. London: King's Fund.

Lewis, J. (2002) 'Research and Development in Social Care: Governance and Good Practice', *Research, Policy and Planning*, 20: 1, pp. 3–10.

Macdonald, G. (1997) 'Social Work Research: the State We're In', *Journal of Interprofessional Care*, 11: 1, pp. 57–65.

Milewa, T., Dowsell, G. and Harrison, S. (2002) 'Partnerships, Power and the "New" Politics of Community Participation in British Health Care', *Social Policy & Administration*, 36: 7, pp. 796–809.

National Institute for Social Work (2000) ESRC-funded seminar series 'Theorising Social Work Research'. http://www.elsc.org.uk/social-careresource/tswr/tswrindex.htm

Parton, N. (1999) 'Social Work: What Kinds of Knowledge?' Paper presented to the ESRC seminar series 'Theorising Social Work Research', Brunel University, 26.5.99.

Available electronically at http://www.elsc.org.uk.socialcareresource/tswr/seminar1/parton.htm

Pawson, R. and Tilley, N. (1997) *Realistic Evaluation*. London: Sage.

Randall, J. (2002) 'The Practice-Research Relationship: a Case of Ambivalent Attachment?' *Journal of Social Work*, 2: 1, pp. 105–122.

Shaw, I. (1999) *Qualitative Evaluation*. London: Sage.

Shaw, I. and Shaw, A. (1997) 'Keeping Social Work Honest: Evaluating as Profession and Practice', *British Journal of Social Work*, 27, pp. 847–869.

Sheldon, M.E.P. (1978) 'Theory and Practice in Social Work: a Re-examination of a Tenuous Relationship', *British Journal of Social Work*, 8: 1, pp. 1–22.

Sheldon, B. (1998) 'Evidence-based social services: prospects and problems', *Research, Policy and Planning*, 16: 2.

Sheldon, B. and MacDonald, G. (1999) *Research and Practice in Social Care: Mind the Gap*, Exeter: Centre for Evidence-Based Social Services.

Sheldon, B. et al (1999) *Prospects for Evidence-Based Social Care: an Empirical Study*. Exeter: Centre for Evidence-Based Social Services.

Sheppard, M., Newstead, S., Di Caccavo, A. and Ryan, K. (2000) 'Reflexivity and the Development of Process Knowledge in Social Work: a Classification and Empirical Study', *British Journal of Social Work*, 30, pp. 465–488.

Silverman, D. (1993) *Interpreting Qualitative Data*, London: Sage.

Social Care Institute for Excellence (2003) Media release 25 March 2003.

'UK experts win SCIE tender to look at how social care staff use research at work'.

Social Service Inspectorate (2003) *Modern Social Services: a Commitment to the Future*. Annual Report, 2002–3. Available electronically at http://www.doh.gov.uk/ssi/ciann-12.htm

Social Service Inspectorate & Audit Commission (2002) *Getting the Best from Best Value*. Department of Health: London. C (2202)2. www.doh.gov.uk/ssi/gettingbestvalue.htm

Talbot, C. (2000) 'Performing "Performance" – a Comedy in Five Acts'. *Public Money & Management*, Oct–Dec 2000, pp. 63–68.

Turner, M. (1998) *Shaping Our Lives Project Report*, October 1998. London: National Institute for Social Work. Available electronically at http://www.shapingourlives.org.uk/perspectives.htm

Webb, S. (2001) 'Some Considerations on the Validity of Evidence-based Practice in Social Work', *British Journal of Social Work*, 31, pp. 57–80.

Williams, F. (2000) 'Principles of Recognition and Respect in Welfare', in G. Lewis et al (eds) *Rethinking Social Policy*. London: Sage.

Williams, M. (2000) *Science and Social Science*. London: Routledge.

10

Listening to 'Quiet' Voices

Shirley McIver

Introduction

It is only when considering groups of people missed by the majority of studies of health service users views that the current reliance on methods requiring high levels of literacy becomes apparent. Questionnaire surveys, focus group discussions and meetings are three of the approaches adopted most widely, but these all demand highly developed skills in written and spoken English. This chapter aims to examine ways to incorporate the views of people who have communication difficulties in service planning and evaluation.

One of the reasons standard market research methods are usually adopted is the common practice of defining patients as 'service users' or 'consumers of services' rather than partners with the mutual aim of health improvement or symptom relief. The terms 'user' and 'carer' are adopted in this chapter because they are more easily understood and less unwieldy than 'partner' or 'co-producer of health' but an active partnership rather than a market based consumer relationship is implied.

The chapter will examine methods for listening and taking account of the views of those who have some degree of difficulty in expressing themselves through the medium of the English language. Four groups of people will be examined:

i)   Children
ii) People with learning difficulties
iii) Elderly people with dementia
iv) Ethnic minorities whose first language is not English

Each of these groups will be looked at in turn, considering first the policy context before providing examples of methods used and a summary of the key points.

Paying attention to groups missed by these methods is beneficial for a number of reasons. Some are obvious – to address inequalities in opportunities for 'having a voice' and to make sure that services are meeting the needs of minority groups – but there are also less well-recognised effects. Larger numbers of people are likely to benefit from the development and use of methods that do not rely as heavily on good literacy skills. Research methods often suit the researcher and the organisation rather than the user. This can be for reasons of cost, convenience or familiarity, but may also be because they are tried and tested methods that produce reliable data that is accepted as evidence.

It is no wonder that health service practitioners and researchers are hesitant about finding out the views of those with undeveloped or restricted literacy. Research on these perspectives has until recently been difficult to find, and methods have not been widely publicised, appear to require special skills, and produce information of unknown validity and reliability.

This is especially the case where involving users with restricted literacy in planning and evaluating services is concerned because issues such as the representativeness of those involved, marginalisation, and the impact of the researcher on views can be important. However this hesitancy can also have an effect at the individual level where it is sometimes an easier option to miss these users out of decisions, or to involve carers in treatment decisions instead.

Children

The UK health and social care policy context for involving children changed quite significantly during the 1990s. There has been the impact of the UN Convention on the Rights of the Child (1989), the 1989 Children Act and several other changes in legislation affecting children, including the 2000 Child Leaving Care Act, the 2001 Care Standards Act and the 2002 Adoption and Children Bill. Department of Health policy initiatives in health and social care have promoted the involvement of children in decisions. A Children's Taskforce was set up in 2000 with the aim of developing a National Service Framework for Children that will set new national standards across the NHS and social services. A Children's Rights Director was established in 2001 to safeguard vulnerable children living in children's homes. A National Clinical Director for Children was also appointed in 2001 to ensure that services meet the particular needs of children.

This activity has been accompanied by both the greater involvement of children in Department of Health initiatives and an increase in the publication of guidance on involving children. Initiatives include a national reference group of children and young people established by the Department of Health and the National Children's Bureau to inform the Quality Protects programme in England; a Young People in Consultation Project run by the National Children's Bureau and funded by the Teenage Pregnancy Unit to inform the development of policy on teenage pregnancy; and young people's Listening and Responding Teams involved in a number of local authority inspections.

The Department of Health has produced an action plan for involving children and young people (*Listening, Hearing and Responding, 2002*), and guidance on involvement from the Quality Protects Programme (*Research Briefing 3 – Young People's Participation, 2000*). Training resources have been developed including *Total Respect (2000)*, a training pack for local authority social services staff and councillors, that aims to increase understanding of the need for children's participation in decisions. A number of voluntary sector organisations focused on children have also published training resources including Children's Rights Officers and Advocates (CROA) and The Children's Society.

Children, in common with all the groups examined in this chapter, can and will communicate. The main issue is the extent to which they are able to do so in a way that is understandable to the majority of people working in health and social care. There are also a number of other issues that need to be taken into account: their vulnerability, the extent to which they are able to focus attention on a subject, their understanding and experience, and their ability to make decisions. However none of these issues is exclusive to children and most people will be affected to a greater or lesser degree when they are sick or in pain. Given this situation and the fact that children will vary a great deal in literacy levels, it is probably most useful to consider an extreme case, that of autistic children. If there are ways of communicating with children in this category, then it will provide a baseline.

Research involving children with minimal or no speech has often focused on their communication deficiencies but a study by Potter and Whittaker (2001) explored the way children in this category communicated and how the environment could enable them. This study involved 18 children with an average age of 4.5 years who had a medical diagnosis of autism and minimal or no speech. They were observed and video-taped while engaged in a range of everyday activities at special schools. Interviews were carried out with five teachers and four speech and language therapists who worked with the children.

The study found that the children communicated spontaneously in non-conventional ways such as 'physical manipulation' (eg taking an adult's hand over to a desired object), and 're-enactment' (repeating part of an activity as a signal for it to be continued). Some of the children had been taught more conventional ways, such as pointing. A key point made by the study was the importance of using an approach that minimised speech because the children experienced extreme difficulty in understanding it. Many of them withdrew from social interaction when speech was used.

By using a combination of non-verbal communication, such as play, imitation of the child, and bursts of activity with frequent pauses, which allowed time for the child to respond, communication was encouraged. The pauses were particularly important as usually adults did not allow time for the children to respond but tended to verbally prompt them with questions.

This study illustrates the importance of play in getting children's views. Activities and exercises that hold a child's attention and rely on pictures and objects rather than writing are useful when combined with non-verbal ways of expressing preferences such as pointing, moving objects, sorting cards, drawing or drama.

Can the children's views gathered during these exercises be valid and reliable? This is quite possible if the material and the process are standardised so that each child is presented with the same experience and responses are recorded in the same way.

Even when more typical methods are used with children, such as panels and forums, interviews, questionnaires, and diaries, the basic principle of the importance of play in the life of children should be taken into account. These methods need to be adapted to suit the child or young person if they are to be successful.

An example of what can happen when methods are not specifically adapted to suit the needs of children and young people is provided by Barnes (1999). She evaluated two citizens' juries (see chapter 6 for further information about this method), one of which was commissioned by the Millennium Debate of the Age in Swansea and involved young people aged between 15 and 16. This jury resulted in less discussion amongst jurors, indeed the facilitators ended up trying to encourage debate:

> '...*the process often had the characteristics of a question and answer session, with the facilitators seeking to engage jurors by asking them questions which prompted little debate.' (p. iii)*.

This led the researcher to state:

> '*The nature of the deliberative process which developed in the Swansea jury suggests that the model was not the most appropriate way of exploring the ideas and views of young people.' (p. vii)*.

One of the best ways to ensure that the methods adopted suit the needs of children and young people is to involve them in the research process itself. An example of this is the 'Ask Us' programme, a multi-media consultation on children's services led by The Children's Society. This involved over 200 disabled children and young people in England aged between 4 and 24 years old. Some did not use speech or sign language.

Six projects were run by the Children's Society, each provided with a budget to allow flexibility. The projects included:

i)   Young people as researchers working on specific topics
ii) Young people asking other young people for their views

iii) Creative workshops with drama, animation, art and music
iv) Song-writing and using recording studios
v) Puppetry
vi) Video diaries
vii) Discussions led by young people
viii) Leisure activities and visits

The lessons learned from this programme of activities included:

> *'Given appropriate tools and support, all children, including those who were labelled as having 'severe or profound disabilities' and 'challenging behaviour' were able to express their views, wishes and feeling.' (www.jrf.org.uk/knowledge/findings/socialcare/741.asp accessed 10.6.2003)*

Greater involvement in the design and running of the project, plus preparation and training are probably the reasons why a young people's citizens' jury organised by Cambridge City Council was more successful than the one commissioned by the Millenium Debate of the Age and led to the Council winning the IPPR/Guardian Public Involvement Award for 2000. This jury was part of a three stage project that involved a survey, which gathered the views of almost 700 young people, two half day meetings with 40 young people, and the jury involving 15 young people. Jurors received training from two youth workers and participated in exercises to allow them to develop skills in questioning witnesses and processing information. A video made by young people was used as evidence in addition to the findings from focus group discussions (IPPR, 2000).

Another feature of successful projects is the use of a multi-method approach. This allows children to participate in the way that appeals to them. A good example of this, and of the involvement of young people at all stages, is the work of the Office of the Children's Rights Commissioner for London which is campaigning for a Children's Rights Commissioner for England. This organisation has an Advisory Board of children who were recruited through leaflets sent to youth related organisations asking children to apply. The members of the Board were given training and they helped write job descriptions and recruit staff. Meetings take place once a month and these include child-friendly papers and activities.

The Advisory Board designed and distributed 5000 child friendly questionnaires, and two groups of children were also trained to act as researchers on two London estates. Meetings with young people took place in many different settings, resulting in consultation with 3000 children in London. The result was a report that became the basis of the *State of London's Children Report* published in September 2001. Three members of the Advisory Board were also on the Steering Group for the Children's Strategy for London (IPPR, 2001)

In sum, during the 1990s, as government policy has increasingly emphasised the need to listen to children's perspectives on issues that affect them, there have been a number of very successful projects. A consensus on good practice in involving children has emerged and guidance based on lessons learned from these projects is now available. The following are key points:

i)   Involve children from the beginning so that the design incorporates their views
ii)   Children need training and support to help them get involved in research and project planning and design
iii) Methods used to capture adults' views, such as questionnaires, focus groups and citizens' juries can work with children but they need to be adapted to suit their needs
iv)   Play is extremely important so methods that incorporate play principles and involve activities not too dependent on literacy, such as art, video and drama, usually work well
v)   A multi-method approach enabling children to take part at a time, place and way that suits them, is a good strategy
vi)   A systematic approach, project planning, and training for those involved so that good practice in recording and analysing information is followed will help to ensure that data collected is valid and reliable.

People with learning disabilities

Over the past 25 years, policy in the health and social care field relating to people with learning disabilities has undergone considerable change. The name for people with a life-long condition that 'reduces a person's ability to understand new or complex information, to learn new skills and to cope with life independently' (King's Fund, 1999) has also changed from mental handicap to learning difficulty or learning disability. In the 1960s, the majority with this condition were cared for in long-stay hospitals isolated from society. Most of these institutions have now closed and residents live in hostels, shared houses or flats, with responsibility shifting from health to social services. This change has been accompanied by an increasing recognition that people with learning disabilities can and should make their voices heard.

Pressure groups campaigning to end discrimination against people with learning disabilities have contributed to this change. The People First movement, which attempted to coordinate the development of the self-advocacy movement started in Oregon in 1974 and became established in England about ten years later (Armstrong, 2002). The social model of disability has also been influential in raising awareness about the ways in which society disables people rather than any mental impairment or limitation. However this model is not generally widespread amongst people working in the health and social care sectors and consequently advocates and self-advocacy groups can be treated with suspicion and a lack of understanding (Armstrong, 2002).

Many local authorities are moving towards providing support to enable more people to find their own accommodation, employment, leisure and education but many still experience exclusion from 'an ordinary life' and also often lack access to health care, despite the fact that they suffer more than average from conditions such as mental illness, epilepsy, heart disease, weight gain, and hearing loss (King's Fund, 1999)

In March 2001, the Department of Health issued a White Paper *Valuing People: A new strategy for learning disability in the 21st century*. This emphasises the need for a fundamental shift in the way public services are provided if people with learning disabilities are to move to full citizenship. The four key principles underlying the White Paper are rights, independence, choice and inclusion. Listening to the views of people with learning disabilities and involving them in decisions that affect them are an important part of the proposals but those providing services to people with learning disabilities are frequently unsure about how they can carry this out. This often leads to an assumption that an individual is incapable of making a choice. (Values into Action, 1999)

Take a routine health check such as a cervical smear test for example. There is a low incidence of uptake of cervical screening among women with learning disabilities (DoH, 2001). This is thought to be due to a combination of factors including a lack of literacy skills, anxiety at the procedure, the woman's capacity to consent, and assumptions that women with learning disabilities are sexually inactive (Broughton, 2002). A project organised by Horizon NHS Trust showed that it was possible to provide cervical screening for women with learning disabilities provided they were informed and prepared by carers who were knowledgeable about the procedure (Shaughnessy, 1999).

Two key points relating to this process are the provision of information and support to enable the person to make a decision. Although not all people with learning disabilities can read, many can interpret pictures or a combination of words and pictures. The Valuing People website has been designed with help from advisers with learning disabilities and provides a good example of how information can be conveyed in a more accessible way (www.doh.gov.uk/vpst).

Research carried out by Values into Action (VIA) explored the decision making process in more detail in order to determine the kind of support people with learning disabilities need in order to make decisions and be in control of their life. The researchers conducted semi-structured interviews and observations with 17 people with high support needs living in nine different homes in England and Scotland. They also carried out interviews and discussions with staff, family and friends of the people (VIA, 2001).

They found that sometimes staff or family members doubted the individual's ability to communicate and express preference and these assumptions were not only likely to be inaccurate but they also became self-fulfilling. However, the researchers found that with the right kind of support everyone could make choices. A number of factors were found to be important for this to happen. These included:

i)   Seeing decision making as a process involving everyone, not a 'test' that the individual had to pass.
ii) Involving individuals in choice and decision-making at all times
iii) Involving the individual's supporters (friends, peers, family, advocates, staff etc) in supporting the individual to make decisions

iv) Routinely using imaginative and effective ways to communicate
v) Using simple, appropriate language and suitable environments
vi) Collaborating as a team and taking collective responsibility for recording evidence of choices
vii) Recording the decision making process in detail, using imaginative methods (pictures, photographs etc)
viii) Maximising the range of options available to people
ix) Reviewing decisions and outcomes, and the individual's satisfaction with them

The researchers found that apart from the attitudes of those caring for the people in the study, a number of structural factors also limited choice and control. These included poor staffing levels that gave staff little time to develop communication and relationships with individuals; fixed organisational procedures, around money for example; an organisational culture that inhibited staff from taking risks; lack of staff training and lack of independent advocacy (VIA, 2001)

There are many examples of people with learning disabilities being involved in the monitoring and evaluation of services and in health and social care research more generally. The Norah Fry Research Centre at the University of Bristol has been one of the leaders in developing this kind of participatory approach. In one project on gender issues that aimed to discover people's perceptions in relation to gender and identify areas of service provision where it was important to take gender into account, service users with learning disabilities planned and conducted the research project and reported the findings (Townsley, 2000).

Eleven people from a resource and activity centre in Avon were involved in the project, supported by their group worker and a researcher. They decided to carry out a questionnaire survey, designed the questionnaire and sent out 400 copies to adults with learning disabilities. The questionnaire included questions accompanied by a picture or symbol that encapsulated the main message and 162 responses were received. The project workers then presented the findings at two seminars (Townsley, 2000).

Another source of examples of projects are the many self-advocacy groups that have developed. These are usually also able to provide training for both staff and people with learning disabilities. However it is important that the history and context of many of these groups is taken into consideration so that health and social care staff will be able to develop an understanding of how they can work in partnership with them. A good example is *Advocacy in Action* which was set up in 1988 as a worker collective by a group of learning disabled and non-disabled people in Nottingham. This group initially experienced considerable resistance to their work so when they achieved success by winning the 'Social Work Today' award for Innovation in Community Care in 1990 they were not too happy to welcome the statutory organisations that suddenly seemed interested in them:

> *'We had learned to manage without friends and we had learned the value and potential of ourselves. And this was how we got our "challenging behaviour" label.' (Advocacy in Action, no date).*

Unless those working in the health and social care sector are prepared to accept a degree of challenge to their preconceptions, they are likely to find partnerships with self-advocacy groups difficult. It would be a good idea to make sure that staff are introduced to likely areas of conflict through awareness raising sessions that help them to examine their attitudes and beliefs.

In sum, although government policy, particularly the 2001 White Paper *Valuing People*, has become more explicit about extending democratic rights such as 'choice' and 'voice' to people with learning disabilities, this has not yet made the kind of impact on the lives of most people that pressure groups would like to see. There are several reasons for this including inadequate staffing levels resulting in lack of staff time as well as other environmental factors such as historically rigid procedures and lack of resources, but also the attitudes of staff and carers and lack of knowledge about how to support people to be involved. There is a very well developed knowledge base about the ways that people with learning disabilities can be supported to provide their views and many examples of research projects that involve them at all stages. The following are key points:

i) Support to communicate and make decisions should be part of everyday activities so that providing views is not a new or unusual activity

ii) Staff and carers should assume that people with learning disabilities can be involved in planning and evaluating services

iii) They should be involved in all aspects of the research process in order to make sure that methods are user friendly
iv) A multi-media approach to collecting and recording views should be adopted, making use of clear simple language, pictures and symbols, large print, video and audiotapes, photographs, drama, art, and activities.
v) Advocates can help as role models and by providing examples

People with dementia

It is currently estimated that approximately 700,000 people in the UK have dementia, with 18,500 of these being under 65. The annual cost to the NHS in England of caring for people with Alzheimer's disease was estimated at over £1 billion in 1993 (Milne and Lingard, 2001; DoH, 2001; Alzheimer's Society, 2003). This constitutes a large group of users of health and social care yet it is a group whose views are not usually heard. People with dementia are probably the least likely to be asked for their views because their communication problems seem to be based upon the disintegration and fragmentation of the personality.

In line with social policy concerning the other groups of vulnerable people included in this chapter, there have been recent changes. In 1993, the World Health Organisation defined dementia as:

> 'A syndrome due to disease of the brain, usually of a chronic or progressive nature in which there is an impairment of multiple higher cortical functions, including memory, thinking, orientation, comprehension, calculation, learning capacity, language and judgement. Consciousness is not clouded. The cognitive impairments are commonly accompanied by and occasionally preceded by deterioration in emotional control, social behaviour or motivation'.

As social science perspectives on health and illness have gradually gained ground, this definition has been seen as overly biomedical. It omits the social context of the condition, failing to recognise that similar symptoms may be interpreted and responded to differently depending on the culture.

During the 1990s an alternative view has emerged of dementia as a socially embedded condition. This takes a person-centred approach that draws on a social disability rather than medical model (Alzheimer's Society, 2003). Health and social care policy has started to reflect this view and there is an increasing emphasis on individualised care. For example the National Service Framework for Older People, standard seven, relates to mental health in older people and includes requirements for support and information for older people with mental health problems and their carers as well as culturally appropriate services for ethnic minorities.

There is still resistance to routinely involving service users with dementia in decisions however. One of the problems is the law on mental capacity. Current law in England states that a person either has capacity to make decisions or they are mentally incapable. If they are deemed incapable they and their carers need not be consulted about decisions as health and social care professionals can make decisions 'in the best interests of the person'. Dementia affects different people in different ways and in reality the ability to make decisions is not 'all or nothing'. This legal situation also has an impact on other vulnerable groups, such as people with learning disabilities, severe mental health problems or autism.

The law has recently been changed in Scotland to enable people to make their own decisions for as long as possible and a new draft mental incapacity bill was announced for England in 2003. If legislation is changed it is likely to increase pressure on health and social care workers to find out the views of people with dementia.

Although not widely appreciated, research incorporating the views of service users with dementia has taken place for more than ten years. For example, the National Consumer Council interviewed elderly people with dementia and their carers living at home, in a study looking at their home care needs (NCC, 1990). This study used a skilled interviewer who found she had to spend time getting to know and gaining the trust of the interviewees, as well as by returning to questions on different occasions.

More recently a project by Kate Allan had the aim of identifying ways in which care staff could develop approaches to consultation with people with dementia (Allan, 2001). She involved 31 people with dementia and 40 staff in 10 services including day, residential and long-term nursing care. The study was exploratory and the researcher considered the area largely undeveloped. Her research approach was action oriented in that she helped staff to reflect on their practice and refine it.

Allan found that consultation could take place in many ways, including:

- Verbally during intimate care
- During trips out and recreational pursuits
- At dedicated times using pictures or other visual stimuli
- By observing non-verbal reactions

One of the most important findings was that indirect approaches seemed to work best. That is where questions were not direct and personal and which allowed the service user the maximum degree of control over what was spoken about. For example, showing them a picture of a person with whom they might identify and asking them to speculate on what they might think or feel about aspects of a service.

The researcher also found that staff involved in the project valued the time provided for discussing and reflecting on their experiences. This gave them new insights and ideas about what worked. Many staff also kept written notes and found these useful as a way of reflecting on the work, remembering points, and sharing experiences with other staff. Some also made audio recordings of their conversations with service users and these tapes enabled them to learn about their own communication style and that of the service user.

Experience of involving people with dementia in activities such as research, service planning and evaluation is increasing, particularly in the voluntary sector. The Alzheimer's Society, for example, won the IPPR/Guardian Public Involvement in the Health Sector award in 2001 for its involvement of users in all aspects of its research programme. The Society recruited 150 volunteers who had experience of dementia either personally or as a carer onto a Consumer Network. This is involved in all aspects of its research programme including strategy setting, commissioning, grant application reviewing, grant awards, project management, dissemination and implementation. Members of the network receive a monthly newsletter, have access to a dedicated website and hold regular regional meetings (IPPR, 2001)

In sum, attitudes to dementia are changing and a social disability model that incorporates an understanding of the ways in which different environments can contribute to the symptoms of the condition is gaining ground in the health and social care field. This emphasises the value of communication in helping to slow down the progress of the condition and involving service users in decisions is an important element of communication.

Despite this change in attitude, progress on getting the views of dementia sufferers has been slow. This is partly because the present law on capacity to consent operates in an 'all or nothing' way and this works against involving people as much as possible. A contributing factor is that members of staff often lack the time and the training to communicate with users. Methods and approaches to involving this group are in the early stages of development but exploratory research suggests that the following are key points:

i)   Opportunities should be taken to ask people for their views during everyday activities
ii) A variety of approaches should be adopted including the use of stimuli such as pictures, photographs, television, drama, singing and reminiscence.
iii) An indirect approach to questions seems to work well, such as asking what a person in a picture might think about services
iv) Users and carers should be involved in all aspects of the research process in order to make sure that methods are user friendly

Ethnic minorities whose first language is not English

The UK policy context for involving black and minority ethnic people is that of addressing inequalities. This includes inequalities in health outcomes as well as inequalities in access to services. Public authorities have an explicit duty to promote race equality following the Race Relations (Amendment) Act 2000. This includes general duties relating to the elimination of racial discrimination, promoting equality of opportunity and promoting good race relations between people of different racial groups, and specific duties applicable to both employment and service delivery.

Reducing health inequalities is one of the government's key priorities for the NHS in the Priorities and Planning Framework for

2003–2006. This sets out the need to identify a single set of local priorities with partners, supported by tools such as equity audits and in response to community needs.

There are a number of important aspects to improving access to services for ethnic minorities. These include providing better information, facilitating communication and developing culturally sensitive services. The involvement of ethnic minorities at both the individual level of treatment and care and the collective level of service planning, design and evaluation is crucial.

Research has demonstrated that the NHS in particular does not have a good record for involving ethnic minorities in the planning and evaluation of services or involving non-English speakers in treatment decisions. Looking first at the collective level, a review of methods for obtaining the views of black users of health services found that response rates to questionnaire surveys were often low, even when handed out at community events (McIver, 1994). The most successful research methods were found to be structured or semi-structured interviews conducted by bilingual interviewers, and focus group discussions facilitated by bilingual researchers. It was important that interview schedules and discussion checklists were constructed with the help of members of the communities concerned, due to the difficulty of translating concepts into another cultural context (McIver, 1994).

Informal methods, such as consultation meetings and forums, also worked well but the key to success was working closely with the relevant ethnic minority communities, taking care to involve different subgroups and working with them on a long term rather than 'one off' basis (McIver, 1994). There can be different priorities for different subgroups and a failure to address priorities can inhibit their involvement. For example a study examining ways to involve black disabled people found that the provision of an accessible and comfortable venue was their priority, yet this aspect was rated eighth by professionals and so was frequently neglected (Evans and Banton, 2001).

In many studies of ethnic minority views about health services, difficulties in communication emerge as the most important issue. For example:

> 'The single most important factor which came out spontaneously among respondents whose first language was not English, was the language barriers they faced when interacting with health and social care professionals...' (Swarup, 1993, p. 41)

The best way of tackling this issue is obviously to make interpreters and bilingual advocates available so that users can understand the risks and benefits of treatment and can make informed
decisions. However, with training, health and social care workers
can improve the situation a great deal. Guidance on how to communicate across a language barrier can be found in Henley (1986,
88) and National Extension College (1991). For example:

i)   Speak slowly and clearly but do not raise your voice
ii) Choose words the patient is likely to know
iii) Use pictures or mime
iv) Think before you speak, and break the topic down into
     logical steps
v)   Signal when you change the subject
vi) Try to learn a few words in the patient's language, such as
     'yes' and 'no'
vii) Keep a phrase book
viii) Use red cross language cards

Interpretation services are clearly essential in aiding communication and helping minority ethnic people to give their views.
Advocacy services have also been found to be useful in developing
involvement at both the individual and collective levels but even
here, culturally inappropriate services can limit access. A study
exploring the need for advocacy services for black and minority
ethnic mental health service users in Trent and Yorkshire, for
example, found that individual and community advocacy was considered necessary to enable communities to engage in the development of new and more culturally appropriate services. Yet this
study found that mainstream advocacy services did not promote
ways of empowering black service users and consequently few
black service users were in contact with the services. Black mental
health users and carers had different views from the mainstream
on what they wanted out of an advocacy service. Contrary to the
ideals of self-advocacy they preferred to have paid professional
advocates and wanted people who reflected their ethnicity and
gender and could understand their views and experiences. Shared
cultural identity was essential (Rai-Atkins et al, 2002).

In sum, promoting racial equality and addressing inequalities in
health outcomes and access to services are government priorities.

This means that the involvement of black and minority service users will have an increasingly high profile. Studies of health service users views generally receive a poor response from black and minority groups unless methods are designed specifically to capture their views. At the individual level, patients are unable to be involved in decisions about treatment and care unless interpreting services and advocates are made widely available and health and social care workers follow good practice guidelines in communicating across a language barrier. Black and minority groups need to be involved in the planning and design of all services if they are to be culturally appropriate. There are many examples of projects where black and minority communities have been successfully involved. Some of the factors contributing to effective engagement include:

i)   Building long term partnerships with community groups
ii) Engaging bilingual researchers and project workers
iii) Making sure that the needs and priorities of different sub-groups of black and minority people are taken into account
iv) Training staff in how to communicate across a language barrier
v)   Employing interpreters and advocates

Conclusions

This examination of research on involvement methods for four different groups of users who are not often included in studies of users views has revealed many similarities. Although the policy context for each is different, there are a number of common issues and what has been found to be effective in involving these groups is also frequently the same.

The main commonality between the different groups is the issue of inequality. There are questions about the extent to which they have received equal rights and equal access to services, and this has resulted in poorer health outcomes in some cases. All have been discriminated against on age, race or mental capacity grounds. All these groups face similar issues involving various degrees of stereotyping by health care workers, organisational discrimination and cultural assumptions about capacity.

Inequality, particular the focus of this chapter which is on inequality of opportunity to have a 'voice' in health and social care services, marks these groups out as different, but this is a difference of degree rather than kind. Indeed many of the factors that have been identified as contributing to effective involvement for these groups constitute good practice in involving users more generally.

In conclusion, health and social care institutions have for some time recognised that the involvement of service users in care decisions, service planning and evaluation can lead to more appropriate and effective services. Until recently involvement has been limited to groups that can respond to the rather narrow range of research methods and approaches adopted. The time has come to take the lead from research involving traditionally excluded groups and develop processes that enable much wider participation.

References

Armstrong, D. (2002) The politics of self advocacy and people with learning difficulties, *Policy and Politics*, 30(3): 333–345.

Advocacy in Action (no date) *Inclusive and empowered communities 1989–2002 the 'challenging behaviour' years*, from 30 Addison Street, Nottingham, NG1 4HA (0115 9470780).

Alzheimer's Society (2003) Wakefield and Five Towns Young Onset Dementia Project final report (www.alzheimers.org.uk).

Allan, K. (2001) Communication and consultation: Exploring ways for staff to involve people with dementia in developing services, The Policy Press.

Barnes, M. (1999) Building a Deliberative Democracy: An Evaluation of Two Citizens' Juries, Institute for Public Policy Research.

Broughton, S. (2002) A review of the literature: interventions to maximise capacity to consent and reduce anxiety of women with learning disabilities preparing for a cervical smear test, *Health Services Management Research*, 15: 173–185.

Evans, R. and Banton, M. (2001) *Learning from experience: involving black disabled people in shaping services,* Council of Disabled People (Fordsfield, Bury Road, Leamington Spa, Warwickshire, CV1 3HW: 01926 420702).

Henley, A. (1986) Nursing care in a multi-racial society, *Senior Nurse*, 4(2): 18–20.

Henley, A. (1988) *Caring in a multi-racial society*, Bloomsbury Health Authority Department of Community Medicine (copy in King's Fund Centre library).

IPPR (2000) Aiming for Excellence in Public Involvement, The IPPR/Guardian Public Involvement Awards, 2000, Institute for Public Policy Research.

IPPR (2001) *The IPPR/Guardian Public Involvement Awards 2001*, Institute for Public Policy Research.

King's Fund (1999) Briefing: Learning disabilities from care to citizenship, King's Fund, 11–13 Cavendish Square, London, W1M0AN (0171 307 2400; www.kingsfund.org.uk).

Milne, A. and Lingard, J. (2001) Dementia advice and support: a new service initiative, *Journal of Dementia Care*, May/June: 28–30.

McIver, S. (1994) *Obtaining the Views of Black Users of Health Services*, King's Fund Centre for Health Services Development.

National Consumer Council (1990) *Consulting Consumers in the NHS, A Guideline Study*, 20, Grosvenor Gardens, London, SW1W 0DH.

National Extension College (1991) Caring for Everyone: Ensuring Standards of Care for Black and Ethnic Minority Patients, The National Extension College Trust Ltd.

Potter, C. and Whittaker, C. (2001) *Enabling communication in children with autism*, Jessica Kingsley Publishers.

Rai-Atkins Asha et al (2002) Best practice in mental health: Advocacy for African, Caribbean and South Asian communities, The Policy Press.

Swarup, N. (1993) *Equal Voice: Black Communities' Views on Housing, Health and Social Services*, Social Services Research and Information Unit, Portsmouth Polytechnic.

Shaugnessy, P. (1999) Better cervical screening for women with learning disabilities, *Nursing Times*, 3(95): 44–5.

Townsley, R. (2000) Archive – *Avon Calling*, June 5, communitycare.co.uk accessed 17.6.2003.

Values into Action (2001) Who's in control? Decision-making by people with learning difficulties who have high support needs, Oxford House, Derbyshire Street, London E2 6HG.

WHO (World Health Organisation) quoted in Alzheimer's Society (2003) *Wakefield and Five Towns Young Onset Dementia Project final report* (www.alzheimers.org.uk).

11

Taking Account of 'Consumer's' Views: Rapport, Reflexivity and the Subjective Interpretation of Narratives in Qualitative Health Research

Paula Nicolson

Introduction

This chapter examines the extent to which the processes of collection and analysis of data in qualitative research owe their strengths to the *subjective skills* and *experience* of the researcher rather than a rigorous adherence to methodological guidelines (see Chapter 7). It is essential to understand this when investigating 'consumer' views in health and social care. The user, or 'consumer' is defined broadly in this chapter as the patient/client and/or the practitioner, from the standpoint that health and social-care workers are frequently 'consumers' of policy and practice surrounding health-related procedures and technologies.

Qualitative research appears to be widely accepted now as a significant player in the field of health services research (HSR) and health research generally. It is particularly acknowledged as a method for eliciting users' (or 'consumers') views of health and social-care (see Chapter 7).

However a tension exists when qualitative research takes place in the health and clinical arenas where the randomised control trial (RCT) is perceived as the 'gold standard'. This has caused some qualitative researchers to lose their voices to calls from the quantitative health research lobbies for 'validity', 'proof' and 'generalisability'. The result of this is that in many cases qualitative health research has become either a lame-duck, simply providing brief descriptive 'thematic' data that might well have been more convincing, and certainly cheaper to collect, via a survey or structured interview; or it has led researchers towards an emphasis on method over research problem (Chamberlain, 1999) which has also meant impotence (Chapter 7).

In what follows I argue that qualitative researchers need to acknowledge and reclaim their strengths even though these may be at odds with mainstream quantitative research. Qualitative research is different from quantitative research in its aims, objectives and outcomes. Qualitative research reveals the contradictions and paradoxes that define the human condition and as such is brazenly interpretive and subjective. Qualitative methods 'count in' rather than 'control for' the processes and the context in which in-depth data (elicited from conducting focus groups and interviews in particular) are collected and thus is technically, but deliberately, 'biased' (see Nicolson, 2003). The concepts of 'rapport, 'reflexivity' and 'subjectivity' are all closely interconnected in the processes of collecting data (or conducting interviews) and analysing the data. To carry out research in this way *rapport* is essential and that involves enabling the respondents to reflect and also to express their subjective experiences. The interviewer likewise needs to engage with the respondent, reflect *operative reflexively* during the interview and in relation to the data analysis. Qualitative researchers also need to acknowledge and 'count in' and include their subjectivity throughout the whole exercise from identifying the research question and design, conducting the face to face work and in analysing the data.

What qualitative research can do

Qualitative research focusing on the views of health care 'consumers' allows investigators to identify the *quality and complexity* of users' experiences and the *different levels* at which the health care user understands the processes of their health, illness and care. There is a range of other methods (as is apparent from this volume) that are useful for more systematic, less person-centred data collection. Here I draw attention to the special contribution of qualitative research in individual and group interviews focusing on the roles of *rapport, reflexivity and subjectivity* and ways in which understanding and paying attention to these processes provides valuable insights into 'consumer' perspectives on health.

To illustrate my arguments I use examples from in-depth interviews with senior health care workers discussing the impact of political and organisational practices on their working life, which was conducted as part of a study of staff stress in a national study of neonatal intensive care units[1] (NICUs) (Tucker et al, 2001). This was part of a study funded by the English Department of Health, during a period when decisions about the provision of NICU services were being discussed. I also use examples from a focus group study of people who have been diagnosed with chronic bronchitis (Nicolson and Anderson, 2001; 2003) to gain a view of their experiences of the diseases and the health care provision.

Rapport

> An implicit factor of a successful interview is that of good rapport between the participant and the interviewer, but this is a surprisingly ill-defined concept, given its centrality to social science research. Although everyone agrees that rapport is essential, situations that accentuate rapport, such as repeated interviews, have also been seen as problematic methodologically (Mathieson, 1999, 128–9).

Rapport means 'affinity' or 'connection' and most interview manuals cite the need to establish rapport between the interviewer/researcher and interviewee. This immediately raises two methodological considerations. The first that an interview in which 'rapport' needs to be established cannot be 'unbiased'. The second being the assumption that it is the interviewer/expert who has the responsibility for ensuring rapport is established rather than all the participants.

Is rapport 'bias'?

I have found repeatedly that co-researchers in multi-disciplinary teams where the majority are quantitative researchers, question the possibility that an interview has anything specific to offer. The question is posed as to whether anyone will talk frankly about the issues they are to be questioned about – I have been asked this question repeatedly ranging over topics as diverse as the transition to motherhood, the experience of being burgled, domestic abuse and chronic disease. There seems to be a contradictory anxiety among the sceptics that no connection between the participants (i.e. researcher and researched) will be made and thus no data will result. However at the same time there is a fear that if a bond that engages the respondent is made, it will produce data that is 'biased'. In the neonatal study for example my colleagues[2] wondered whether any 'busy health professional' would have the time to talk to me about their role in the organisation. Would in-depth interviews be worthwhile? I was asked repeatedly. As you will see from the examples I have chosen, there was no problem – people (mostly) *do* want to talk about things that impact upon their lives. I have rarely experienced anyone who has agreed to be interviewed being unprepared to talk frankly and at length. In the NICU study for example there were respondents who have started off cynically – 'I'm not sure what I can tell you about ....'. But much of the time this attitude changes as the interview progresses. There are also respondents who clearly have been interviewed so often before that what they tell you is well-rehearsed and regardless of interviewing skills, this type of respondent tries to stick to their 'script'.

Whoever you meet though, you have to establish rapport and the data then becomes more than just the 'facts'. Data includes *the process*es of gathering the facts, feelings, emotions and the context in which all of that is expressed. This process becomes particularly problematic (but also interesting!) when considering the role of electronic interviews and discussion groups as shown in Chapter 8).

Interviewing is a skill that many researchers (particularly those who disdain qualitative research) take for granted. It requires an ability to listen and to have the confidence to follow the reasoning and ideas of the respondents while remaining true to the research inquiry. It also requires the confidence to risk making one-self look foolish sometimes by asking deliberately naïve questions and sometimes making mistakes because you have not fully under-stood the answer. This is a skill. It is difficult to conduct good in-depth semi-structured interviews, but with confidence and practice it is extremely worthwhile.

Responsibility for rapport

It is typically expected that the onus for establishing rapport should be on the researcher because it is s/he who is assumed to have the major investment in the interview 'working' as well as the skills to bring it off. However that is not necessary, particularly when user views are being sought.

As you can see from my interview[3] with 'Michael'[4] there is a level of personal connection between us in which he is making equal effort to create, whereby he reveals important contextual material about himself as a husband and father as well as senior consultant.

> **Michael**: *My problem is that I feel that I am failing in both departments – I am not particularly succeeding in work because I try to get home – and I am not particularly succeeding at home because I am not really that efficient at home – I feel I am doing a mediocre job sometimes I wish I could do a really good job in one.*
>
> **Paula**: *Have you told your wife that – the way you have told me?*
>
> **Michael**: *Yes – we talk a lot – some of it you can't blame on work – she certainly feels that … we are on a bit of a knife edge at the moment – I feel – I hope it works I am optimistic but I just can't seem to manage it all you know – I would love to do a good job here – but if I do a good job here I seem to need to be here all the time – I don't want to be here all the time – I have no desire to ….*

By engaging in this way, both Michael and I immediately got a sense of how he measured himself against his understanding of how these roles fitted into the social structure of the NICU. He evaluated himself and his performance in accordance with standards he saw as being set outside his/himself. He saw these standards as more important for self-evaluation than his own judgments about what is possible for him. His ability and willingness to make a connection enabled me to interpret more of the context of his working environment than if he had provided a list of stresses and strains. That would have had value, but not provide insight into how people make sense of their worlds in the way that this extract reveals.

My understanding of what was happening and what was being discussed in the interview might be different from Michael's or other people reading the extract or the full transcript. However, for rapport to be established the interviewer has to engage with the respondent *on a level apart from the objective collection of 'data'*. It requires a rapid connection on a particular level at which both are comfortable. The respondent *has to want to talk to the interviewer and to tell her/him things they want to know.* This requires complex negotiation. Typically in academic psychology, and other social sciences, perhaps to a lesser extent, the interview process is not *meant* to be a relationship, but a means to extract the 'truth' or 'facts' from the respondent about their attitudes, behaviour or whatever is being studied.

Often the respondents themselves anticipate the interview, keen to ensure rapport with the researcher which enables maximum impact of their accounts. This may mean a level of intimacy as with Michael:

> **Michael**: *I have looked forward to this discussion – there are issues here that I want to sort out.*

Or, as with Walter who is of similar professional status in a different unit, but who has no desire or intention to reveal his *personal* experiences if he can help it. This becomes clear and we both negotiate quickly how far I can go in finding out the level of stress he is dealing with:

> **Paula**: *Why have you chosen this speciality?*

> **Walter**: *Paediatrics with neonatal interest. I qualified in medicine in 19xx, specialised in paediatrics three/four years later and as my time went on I found my specific skills and the area of work I enjoyed related to care of patients and their carers. Neonatology gives by far the most intimate involvement between patients and their carers. You get a much more extended period of inter-involvement*

than you get in any other part of paediatrics. Also I perceive the new born as being amongst the most vulnerable in society and therefore the area of work in which I operate has been developing extensively over the past 15 years, as such we are able to do things now that we couldn't before and there's a lot of excitement generated by that.

Almost immediately we established a rapport in our relationship whereby Walter would talk to me initially only about things he had thought through – possibly in anticipation of my visit. After some negotiation he began to answer my questions, rather than provide what seemed to be a well-rehearsed line, but for the most part he would leave out the reflexive, intimate or underlying personal elements of his experiences. He wants to be clear and impersonal. He focused on what 'we' did.

> **Paula:** *The biggest problem might have been, by the sound of it, the budget combined with a lack of knowledge about the clinical care for the whole region?*
>
> **Walter:** *Exactly right. We were very cautious in doing it, we had to prove to our purchasers that we would not be a) offering an inappropriate level to babies who might actually get better care elsewhere, b) that we were not actually being more expensive than a tertiary unit would be and c) that actually it was in the patients' best interest to do that as opposed to just being an alternative thing. We had to justify the fact that we weren't doing it to improve our units' ego but actually to offer better care for babies.*

He seems to be emphasising that he is a team player. He is also trying, I think, not to be talking about himself or about any thoughts he might have been having about the work and the unit.

Reflexivity

Walter is trying to avoid reflexivity in the context of our interview. But what exactly does that mean? Reflexivity in qualitative research has been defined in a number of ways and for those engaged in collecting in-depth data this continues to be a highly contentious but key concept (see Banister et al, 1994; Nicolson, 2003).

Reflexivity in the research interview requires an analytic approach that accounts for and respects 'the different meanings brought to the research by researcher and volunteer' (Parker in Banister et al, 1994, 14). This assumes the potential for the shared understanding of events or emotional experience, and that the participants experience a sense of meaning *prior* to the research encounter.

Alternatively it may be used to confirm a relativist position, i.e. that *talk* between respondent and interviewer is functional in *creating* what might be seen as individual, prior experiences and meanings. That:

> *taking reflexivity seriously in doing research is marked by a concern for recognising that constructing is a social process, rooted in language, not located inside one's head (Steier, 1991, 5).*

Here I have used the concept in a way that assumes an individual with a biography and a dynamic sense of her/his life's meaning which is produced (and reproduced) in the narrative and analysis of that narrative (Nicolson, 1995; 1998).[5] The interview itself is the site of far more activity than simply the collection of verbal data. It is a reflexive process and one in which a relationship is established and it is this relationship that almost becomes a *third* actor in the research scenario.[6]

To fully understand the way the 'consumer'/user makes sense of the processes of health care it is important to understand how the process of being interviewed, whether individually or in a group, is a dynamic one through which meaning is continually constructed and described. Examples from the two studies indicated the ways in which meaning is constructed, show that the in-depth research interview represents an intervention and how the process of the interview itself generates a biography or history for the participants. This is *valid data* and through counting the reflexive and subjective elements of the engagement between the research participants some important questions can be addressed.

Reflexivity and chronic disease

Quality of life for chronic obstructive pulmonary disease (COPD) 'patients' has been discussed at length (see Nicolson and Anderson, 2003) but scant attention has been paid to the way that people with chronic bronchitis[7] make sense of their condition as a 'patient/consumer' and as a person. The experience of chronic bronchitis involves physical deterioration, emotional distress and a reliance on health care providers both during and in between acute exacerbations. To understand what this might mean for the 'consumer', it is worth re-iterating the point made by Radley (1999) that the individual is *actively* engaged in adaptation to chronic disease. That is they don't just *witness* the deterioration of their health – they try to make sense of it and frequently try to resist it.[8] Whatever the process (adjustment i.e. acceptance of the 'new' self or adaptation i.e. changing affect and behaviour in recognition of what has happened) there is inevitably a sense of loss of self-hood that the respondent negotiates between themselves and their social environment (see Charmaz, 1995).

Qualitative research that takes the reflexive process as data (rather than as something either irrelevant or that has to be controlled for) can gain vital understanding of what it means to be a person with a chronic illness in a way that no other methodology is able to do.

Self, change and reflexivity

The extracts below indicate how the text of the group interviews can reveal the process of adaptation to the losses that occur through the development of chronic disease. For example, a sense of 'blame' in relation to this adaptation can be detected throughout the transcripts, attached to the disease, which is both self-blame and *resistance to being blamed* by others. This sense of blame pervades respondents' *self-esteem*. This blame relates further to a sense of being a 'burden' and of 'self-distaste':

> You get utterly *fed up with yourself*.[9] You *class yourself* as being a *burden*, well that's the way I look at it. (FG4).[10]

This extract suggests an attempt to cast one's self aside, to talk about your 'self' as the object of the phrase/sentence and of scrutiny and criticism, to dismiss and relegate the diseased self (i.e. body *and mind*) to the category of burden, somehow diminishing the negative impact that might affect others and also one's self. This is taken further in the extract below:

> *I think you are <u>causing</u> problems for yourself if you start trying to do things like that* (be active). *I think you have – its like working within your capacity – they are a lot of things you can do – but you <u>have to</u> remember what you can't do and work within that restriction (FG1).*

Again, in this *imperative*, there is an *active sense of resignation* and capitulation. It is important for the person with the disease to act upon the limitations, not to *cause* problems. They need to realise their limitations in order not to burden either self or others by trying to act as if they are fit. They become the 'other' when they have this disease. There is also a clear sense and belief that some 'others' would support this view – not only that of the person with the disease as being a burden, but also to *blame* in some way. The tenor of the phrases used to discuss the self, indicate a harshness of judgment and dismissal of value. The disease is invisible somehow they, the people who are ill, are seen as fraudulent.

> *Yeah, it <u>causes a bit of friction</u> actually – you know my husband will say to me 'what have you been doing all day – why haven't you done this, why haven't you done that'. <u>They don't realise</u> you can't do it you know and as for myself relatively I'm only young and I <u>can't do</u> the things <u>I want to do to</u> be quite honest but <u>they don't understand</u> (FG1).*

There are interesting contradictions implicit in these extracts also. The harshness and imperatives give way to explications of others not 'realising' or 'understanding' the problems of living with chronic bronchitis. Here the self is very much the subject of scrutiny and experience.

However, the ill person is still a *burden*, a situation that is deepened if they are *not yet old* because if you are young there are expectations you have of yourself and that others have of you *that the individual cannot meet*. The frustration in their own incapacities and the impact of perceived and actual outside criticism requires the individual to develop a way of coping with their experience of being in the world.

One method of coping is by separating or splitting the body and the mind: the body that has 'failed' and the mind that, while vulnerable is still the old, capable 'me'.

> ... I think your <u>medical self</u> is <u>not as good</u> as it should be, so when you've done your day whatever you do in the day, go shopping, you sit back on the settee and relax and 'think <u>that's me</u> done today'. If someone rang and said 'are you coming for a pint' and you say 'no', <u>they think</u> you're skint and say 'I'll buy you a beer'. I'm not spending very much I'm probably richer now than I were! (FG 2).

But even this separation of the 'medical' self from the 'me' is vulnerable to the judgment (or perceived judgement) of others. People with the disease recognise that they are a 'burden' to others. The apparent suggestion is that they still experience contradictory messages from others. That indicates that they are not somehow seen as truthful in their behaviours. They are perceived as *poor* or *lazy* (previous extract) and thus *frauds* in some way.

Subjectivity

Everything I have discussed so far includes the concept of subjectivity – qualitative research interviews and the analysis of the data have to include a strong element of subjectivity – in participation, in analysis and interpretation of the interaction at the time of the interaction and the analysis of the resulting texts. It is merely to say that when an interview takes place the participants are conscious at several levels – the practical (here-and-now), the discursive or reflexive and also at an unconscious level. The interviewer, as a participant is not excluded from this process that has been identified and discussed by Giddens:

> All human beings continuously monitor the circumstances of their activities as a feature of doing what they do, and such monitoring always has discursive features (Giddens, 1995, 35).

Human beings have a past, present and expectation of a future that is included in the interview and helps to construct that interview which is key to considering the views of 'consumers'.

The expectation of a visit from a psychologist in the NICU study for example stimulated *reflexive contemplation* in respondents who had specific issues in their stressful work situations that they wanted to resolve. There was a commonality in the way they reflected operate reflexively upon and constructed an analysis of their work and the role of stress in their lives. There was clearly a mutual engagement in the interview *process,* which enabled a *shared construction* of meaning and experience through *reflexivity during, before and after the interview itself.* The groups with chronic bronchitis were inspired by the context in which their condition and how they coped with it was the focus but also something they shared with the others. They thus entered into a consensus-type exercise with their colleagues to explain to me, although quickly and more importantly, to each other, what their experiences felt like to them.

Subjectivity, the interviewer and respondent

The interview itself develops a biography and a history – it exists across time in anticipation of the future encounter, the sense of the present and reflection of the past relationship. Although this is the case in all such encounters, the *biographical and historical* characteristics of the interview. My concern on one level was to ensure data was collected and that it was useful and useable. However I also had concern about the way I would be perceived and concern for the experiences that were being revealed. The nature of the content of both studies involved distress at different levels and this had its impact, upon both me (questioning and listening), and the respondent (telling and remembering). The researcher, almost inevitably and sometimes necessarily, loses track of the fact that they are supposed to be objective researchers – in order to focus on the meaning that events and experiences have upon the lives of the respondent the researcher has to understand and 'get to know' the person they are interviewing. Thus in a real sense I found I cared about the people I was interviewing – some more than others of course – but I developed a feeling of being responsible for their pain and happiness. This was not totally inappropriate given the level of intimate revelations that took place. However such notions are anathema in traditional academic psychology and take a reflexive awareness to recognise.

These points, and the multiple layers surrounding 'reflexivity', 'subjectivity' and 'bias' in the interview are best illustrated through examples. In the extract below Michael, uses the experience of being interviewed to talk *to* and *for* himself (as well as to me) *about* his 'self' and reflect demonstrates reflexivity in relation to the dilemmas he currently seems to face and perceives he faces alone. Not only does he feel he is alone in the working context, but he also has to live up to his sense of how others (he believes) see him. In this example he particularly identifies the 'others' as his parents, and his immediate family of wife and children.

> **Michael:** *My parents see my achievements as being important.. It all looks great to them.. But ... the reality is – when I am asked 'how's work?' – my comment was 'stressful! It's rewarding but stressful'. I wouldn't give it up. I wouldn't resign my job – it's rewarding – but it's stressful. My biggest fear is I suppose is that that stress will take its toll on me and my family – I would feel very cheated if that happened I try to deal with it – I am not bad at it – I have colleagues who hang around until all hours.*

He appears to think he might have to choose between job and family. But if he chooses the latter, he might be a failure in their eyes. His emotional state clearly has an effect on me. The extract continued thus:

> **Paula:** *But that is a way of avoiding facing their families isn't it?*
>
> **Michael:** *Do you think so?*
>
> **Paula:** *Absolutely*

This extract highlights my involvement with his stress and fears about how he (as compared to his colleagues) handles the stress. I have clearly engaged with him in a therapeutic role and I was surprised when subsequently I heard the tape and read the transcript that this had happened. The interview had shifted ground, almost without me realising. Developing rapport through information gathering to an in-depth discussion of Michael's experiences and how he should make sense of them was seamless. I was unclear how or even why it happened. As I write this though several years after the only occasion I met him I still wonder how he managed to resolve the fierce conflicts in his life and hope that our meeting provided some clues to him as how to proceed in tackling his stressful life.

Conclusions

Each encounter between the researcher and respondent, whoever they are, and for however limited the research period, exists in a number of dimensions. Mead's (1934/67) work on the self as 'subject' and 'object' promotes understanding of how an interview is not simply a means of collecting qualitative data on tape and the later analysis of a transcribed text.

Talking to another human being brings individual and shared consciousness into play, and thus reflexive, discursive and unconscious dimensions to the encounter. For the interviewer, there are the multiple anxieties about whether and how the encounter will work – will rapport be established, will the respondent have anything to say and will the questions be well constructed and received?

Thinking about the interview retrospectively brings both the respondent and interviewer more opportunity for reflexivity, although their aims are different. The interviewer will have the tape and transcript to focus on as well as the memory of certain aspects of the encounter and the 'atmosphere'. The respondent will have the memory of their thoughts and emotions generated by the interview process and their relationship with the interviewer.

The processes involved in the in-depth group or individual interview are not (and can never be) neutral, objective and unbiased acts. The interviewer and participant are engaging (or failing to engage) with each other and those processes demand mutual construction of the topics under discussion. The subsequent actions involved in data analysis further reflect demonstrate this process and involve renewed engagement with the data by the researcher.

Taking a qualitative approach to research with users of health and social care, has implications for the researcher as well as the respondent. Conducting a survey, RCT or experiment might be intellectually absorbing and the findings compelling but the focus then is upon the data and the theoretical framework. The in-depth interview requires *commitment* to the lives of the respondents, which frequently 'stay' with the researcher. This aids reflexivity but also results in an on-going construction of the relationship that began with the agreement to be interviewed. It impacts upon the analysis of the data which itself reflects echoes the engagement and reflections reflexivity on around that engagement.

Notes

1. I would like to acknowledge other key members of the neonatal staffing study research team particularly Janet Tucker from the University of Aberdeen and Gareth Parry and Chris McCabe from the University of Sheffield.
2. This was a multi-disciplinary team comprising statisticians, health service researchers, neonatal clinicians and health economists none of whom had experience and few of whom had faith in qualitative research of any kind.
3. From the UKNSS study.
4. All names have been changed.
5. For example in my research interviews I always ended by asking the respondent how they had found the experience. Frequently in response to this or to other questions they will say 'I hadn't seen it that way before..' or 'Talking about it clarified ...'.
6. These ideas were developed initially by symbolic interactionist and phenomenological psychologists in the 1940s–1960s (mostly) in the USA. Some of these ideas influenced the social psychology of the 1970s/80s and the epistemology of contemporary qualitative psychologies, particularly aspects of discourse analysis (e.g. Harre and Secord, 1972)
7. A type of COPD.
8. Nicolson and Anderson (2001) for example, found that people with multiple sclerosis frequently denied the implication of new symptoms even though they were well aware of what future limitations lay in store for them and had identified themselves as having MS.
9. The phrases which represent the core of the interpretation in the analysis are underlined.
10. Four focus groups were conducted and FG1–FG4 are labels used to identify the group.

References

Banister, P., Burman, E., Parker, I., Taylor, M. and Tindall, C. (1994) *Qualitative methods in psychology: A research guide*, Buckingham: Open University Press.

Chamberlain, K. (1999) Using grounded theory in health psychology, in M. Murray and K. Chamberlain (eds) *Qualitative Health Psychology: Theories and Methods*, London: Sage, pp. 183–201.

Charmaz, K. (1995) The body, identity and self: Adapting to impairment, *The Sociological Quarterly*, 36(4) 657–680.

Giddens, A. (1995) Modernity and self-identity: Self and society in the late modern age, Cambridge: Polity.

Harre, R. and Secord, P.F. (1972) *The explanation of social behaviour*, Oxford: Blackwell.

Mathieson, C.M. (1999) Interviewing the ill and the healthy, in M. Murray and K. Chamberlain (eds) *Qualitative Health Psychology: Theories and Methods*, London: Sage, pp. 117–132.

Mead, G.H. (1934) *Mind, Self and Society*, Chicago: University of Chicago Press.

Nicolson, P. (1995) Qualitative research and mental health: Analyzing subjectivity. *Journal of Mental Health*, 4(4): 337–345.

Nicolson, P. (1998) Postnatal Depression: Psychology, Science and the Transition to Motherhood, London: Routledge.

Nicolson, P. (2003) Reflexivity, 'bias' and the in-depth interview: developing shared meanings, in L. Finlay and B. Gough (eds) *Reflexivity: Critical Illustrations for Health and Social Science*, Oxford: Blackwells, pp. 133–145.

Nicolson, P. and Anderson, P. (2001) The psychosocial impact of spasticity-related problems for people with multiple sclerosis: A focus group study, *The Journal of Health Psychology*, 6(5): 551–568.

Nicolson, P. and Anderson, P. (2003) Quality of life, distress and self-esteem: A focus group study of people with chronic bronchitis, *British Journal of Health Psychology* (in press).

Parker, I. (1994) Qualitative research. In: *Qualitative methods in psychology: A research guide*, edited by P. Banister, E. Burman, I. Parker, M. Taylor, and C. Tindall.

Radley, A. (1999) Social realms and the qualities of illness experience, in M. Murray and K. Chamberlain (eds) *Qualitative Health Psychology: Theories and Methods*, London: Sage, 16–30.

Steier, F. (1991) *Research and Reflexivity*, London: Sage.

Tucker, J., Parry, G., McCabe, C.J. and Nicolson, P. et al (2001) *United Kingdom Neonatal Staffing Study*, Health Technology Assessment, Southampton: NHS Executive.

Conclusions: Taking a Critical Perspective: Research Methods and the Role of 'Users' or 'Consumers'

Paula Nicolson and Jennifer Burr

The British National Health Service (NHS) has been the main case study used throughout this book. However the NHS is experiencing a similar series of reforms to health care systems in New Zealand, Canada, Australia and other countries where there are varying degrees of socialised, or mass-insurance health care systems. Therefore, the issues raised in this volume have relevance to health and social care reforms across the Western world. As each writer in this volume has established, defining 'consumer', 'user' and similar terms remains problematic in both policy and research-related discussions and it is our contention that there is a distinct lack of analysis of consumerism in health care. Research *about* health care users' views is abundant, although it is difficult to make a systematic analysis of either its descriptive or its predictive value because:

> ... *health care users' views may be elicited at a multitude of levels. Levels broadly defined included: firstly, the personal views of patients for evaluating local services and in clinical decision-making. Secondly, a further level incorporated 'user groups', more formalised groups with experience of services and with distinct views on those services. Thirdly and finally, users' views could also be expressed in terms of 'public opinion' including views on the need for services and public health concerns. A simpler distinction is that users' views could be differentiated between actual users and potential users (CHePAS, 201, 25).*

The consumer/user seems to exist along a continuum from the 'patient', who has a particular health-related condition, through to the 'ordinary' person who may or may not have the need to call upon health or social care services at some future time. Thus we are all potential 'consumers'. Essentially consumerism is defined in the shift from welfarist principles to neoliberal politics, as outlined in the chapters by Smith and Owen, and in the related shift in emphasis from the state to the individual and the individual's duty to look after their health. And as discussed in the Introduction, consumerism in health care provides an identity and language for claiming rights, but also as consumers, we all experience increasing regulation under the rubric of public health, screening and health promotion activities. In addition, the 1970s political demands for consumer rights were defined through a reduction in medical autonomy rather than through a positive desire to involve 'consumers' in the running of the health service (see Smith in this volume).

The growth in research on users' views has come about mainly because of policy-driven imperatives at the macro and micro levels the background to which has been discussed in the chapters by Elizabeth Clough, Jenny Owen and Graham Smith. Government, for instance, requires consumer participation in service evaluation and ongoing applied research and development. Many of the frustrations for individual researchers and research-informed organisations under the influence of such obligations were brought out in Richard Wilson's chapter and relate particularly to a shortage of time, staff and money and essentially, a lack of coherent strategy for the involvement of consumers, which includes recognition that to do so properly requires extra time, staff and money.

On the micro-level, Government-funded research councils, such as the Medical Research Council (MRC) and the Economic and Social Research Council (ESRC), are equally persuasive in informing the involvement of consumers in research. This is also true for charitable grant giving bodies particularly in the UK, North America and Australia. Academics applying for research funding for applied research in health and social care are 'encouraged' to offer evidence that research will be conducted with some degree of user partnership at the planning, development and implementation stages and users' assessments of research proposals are frequently sought.

Further, the natural 'liberal' tendencies of many of those moti-
vated to research in this area, possibly driven by the potential
their contribution might make to changing and improving the
experience of being a patient, client, user, consumer, or whatever
term is preferred, of caring services feeds into this rhetoric. These
perspectives are illustrated in Chapter 3, where Richard Wilson
presents the views of researchers'. It is tempting to take on board
the rhetoric *that research and health and social care over all will be
improved if we take account of users' views* uncritically. There is no
reason why research into, or designs incorporating consumer perspectives, should be a positive enterprise. It needs to be conducted well. This means, as we have argued throughout, that
appropriate, well planned, and well-resourced research is essential. For this researchers need to understand what they are doing
and why the focus on or involvement of consumers improves the
quality of the design and conduct of the study.

In this book we challenge the assumption that user add-ons
increase the knowledge or evidence base. We have asked questions about the applied definitions of 'users'. We have questioned
how far the outcomes of different research technologies and epis-
temologies enable or disable dialogue between experts and the
public. As Owen suggests, quoting Barnes (2002), if research
methods are to recognise differences in power and diversity of
experience, this requires dramatic changes, both in organisation
and process of research as well as a challenge to the scientific
basis of knowledge production. Drawing on feminist 'standpoint'
theory, Barnes argues that user movements 'expose the particularity of the standpoint from which knowledge is produced (Barnes,
2002, 322 quoted in Owen Chapter 9).

We have emphasised that if the views of the consumer are to be
of any practical use in changing and developing services, it is
important to acknowledge that change cannot happen *merely*
through tapping user views. These views need to be set in the
context of the services, the health or social care 'problem' and
the lives of those who use or will use the services. In other words,
there is absolutely no point in conducting research into users'
views unless there is an agenda for responding to need and expectations and the mechanisms for taking action predicated upon
such views are in place. For example, patient groups have a strong
ethos of involvement in bodies which formulate and implement

health policy. However, there is evidence that different groups are not involved equally in decision-making and that the ability of consumer groups to affect policy agendas is questionable (Allsop, Baggott and Jones, 2002). Furthermore, as McIver in Chapter 10 outlines, there exist a number of groups missed by traditional research methods for a number of reasons including that the majority of studies of health service users require a high degree of literacy. Surveys, focus groups and interviews, all routinely adopted in health service research, all demand highly developed skills in reading, writing and verbal communication. Therefore, groups including children, people with learning difficulties and dementia and ethnic minority groups whose first language is not English are some of the groups often missed by most research methods. The adaptation of methods to suite different groups has not been widely publicised (McIver presents the basics on how to address some of these research inequalities). However, it remains the case that research methods are often developed to suit the researcher and the organisation and therefore, further serve to marginalise groups that already suffer inequality in access to health and social care resources.

What is intriguing, but perhaps unsurprising under the circumstances reiterated in this volume, is that contemporary literature, despite its abundance, for the most part fails to take *a critical position* on the application of this type of research or the significance of seeking user views and participation in research into health and social care. The contributors to this volume have endeavoured to take a critical stance – whether they are *critical of the practice* of employing consumer/user views within the research process or critical of *a particular method/approach* that has been identified or assumed to be appropriate in such a context.

No methods or approaches tell the whole story and neither do they manage to provide representation of what the 'average' patient, consumer, user, member of the public or client might want, need or expect from the caring services. What is clear is that several different methods need to be applied to a specific set of problems, and those problems need to be set in their context. Patient satisfaction surveys, favoured by Government, the NHS and many funding bodies because of their apparent cost-effectiveness are weak in the face of understanding the process of satisfaction with health care (see Collins and Nicolson, 2002). Qualitative data are promoted as being more likely to get to the heart of what people really think. But is this really the case? Qualitative research, hailed as something different, has just as many, albeit different problems as quantitative research and is frequently conducted either without rigour or with so much regard for issues of design, that the strength of qualitative approaches gets lost amid the methodolotary (see Jennifer Burr and Paula Nicolson's chapters).

We have tried to show that good quality research is possible. There are certain rules that need to be understood however, which include awareness that the method should suit the research problem; that research is best carried out by those with the training, expertise and working environment to support it and equally essential is that research needs to be subject to peer scrutiny and available as an evidence base for health and social care providers to consult. It also needs to include the difficulties and what has gone wrong in the research process in order for methods to develop and move forward and generate an evidence base as to whether 'consumer' involvement is a step forward or not.

References

Allsop, J., Baggott, R. and Jones, K. (2002) in Henderson, S. and Petersen, A. (eds) *Consuming Health: The commodification of Health Care*, London: Routledge.

Barnes, M. (2002) 'Bringing difference into deliberation? Disabled people, survivors and local governance', *Policy & Politics*, 30: 3, pp. 319–331.

CHePAS (Consumer Health Psychology at ScHARR) (2001) *Eliciting Users' views of the processes of Health care: A Scoping Study.* The NHS Service Delivery and Organisation (SDO)

Collins, K. and Nicolson, P. (2002) The meaning of 'satisfaction' for people with dermatological problems: re-assessing approaches to qualitative health psychology research, *Journal of Health Psychology*, 7(5): 615–629.

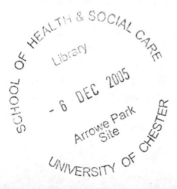

Index